T♥TAL LIVING

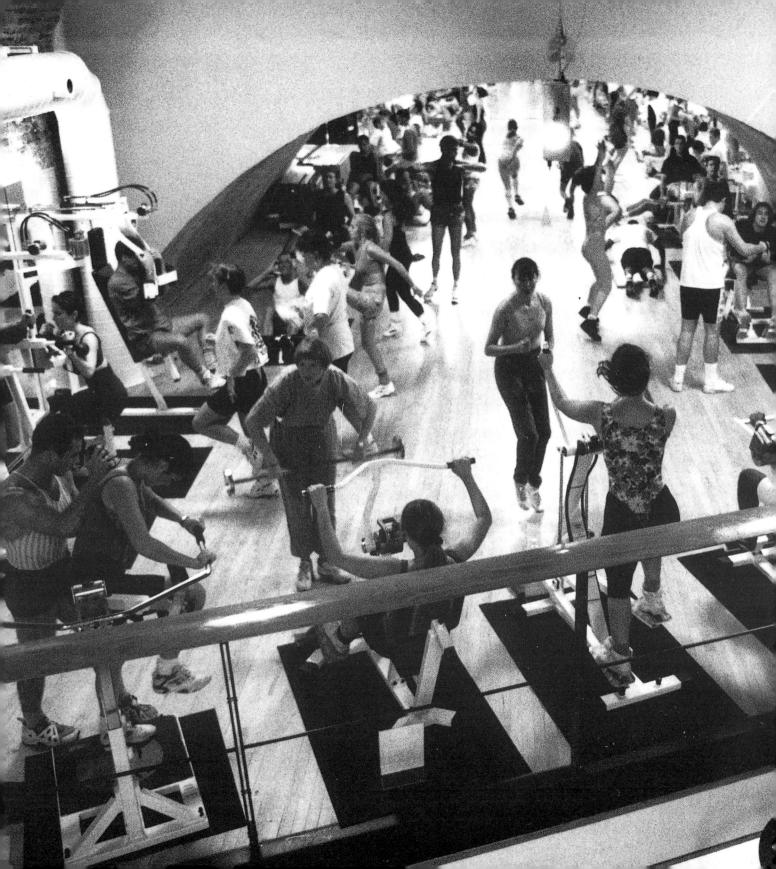

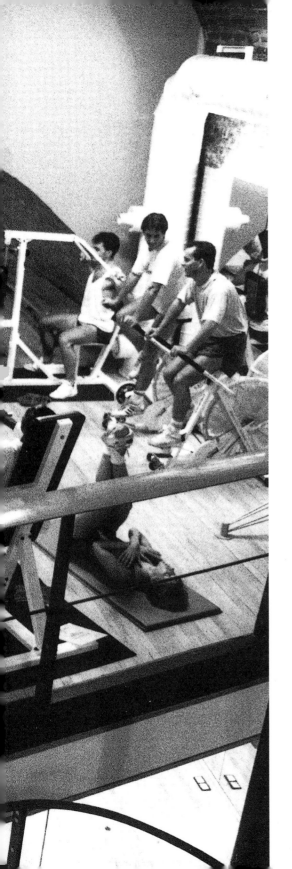

T♥TAL LIVING

For everyone who wants to be
fitter, trimmer and smarter

RON CLARKE

and the team at

CANNONS SPORTS CLUB,

with Dr John Briffa

PAVILION

First published in Great Britain

in 1995 by

Pavilion Books Limited

26 Upper Ground

London SE1 9PD

Text copyright © 1995 by Ron Clarke and Cannons team

For photographic credits, see page 160

The moral right of the author has been asserted

Designed by the Bridgewater Book Company

A CIP catalogue record for this book

is available from the British Library

ISBN 1-85793-4075

Printed and bound in Great Britain

by Butler & Tanner Ltd, Frome and London

10 9 8 7 6 5 4

This book may be ordered by post direct from the publisher.

Please contact the Marketing Department.

TOTAL LIVING

This publication is designed to assist all, from the never-worried-about-my-health-much majority to the ultra-fit fanatic. You are never too old or too young, too fat or too lazy not to be at least curious about how best to improve your current state of health. Nor can you be too knowledgeable.

But, at the same time, it is no textbook. We are not trying to prepare you for a medical degree, Diploma of Nutrition or, for that matter, to be an Olympic athlete.

Each section stands alone, and can be read in any order, but we have assembled them in such a way as to provide the complete picture.

CONTENTS

Forewords by Clive James, Kim Hagger and Sally Gunnell

> *Constant exposure to UVA can improve your aerobic performance (stamina) by up to 20%*

This chapter takes a look at each of the factors known to be important in heart disease and stroke. The relevance of each factor is described, along with advice on the steps that can be taken to reduce the risk of incurring these conditions.

The specific factors which are discussed in relation to heart disease include blood cholesterol, blood pressure, smoking, obesity, diabetes and exercise.

One third of us will develop cancer at some point in our lives. However, many scientists believe that most cancers are preventable.

This chapter describes the factors which may put us at risk of cancer, and gives advice on how we may protect ourselves in the long term.

Although not quite a disease, certainly stress is a product of our lifestyles. It can literally either be a disaster or a joy. Here is how we think you can actually learn to enjoy the pressure.

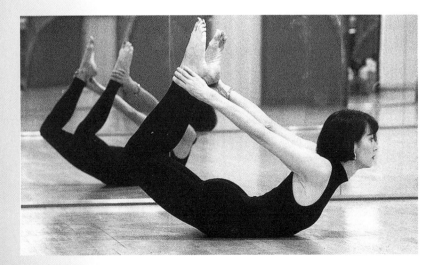

After providing the information you need to know, we now move on to the action sections, chapters where we recommend specific workouts, routines or life changes that will improve your health and well-being significantly. The first of these will surprise many – a chapter on the merits of suntanning. The publicity given to the dangers of ultra-violet radiation (UVA) has been widespread, overwhelming the positive aspects of a healthy suntan. For example, did you know constant exposure to UVA can improve your aerobic performance (stamina) by up to 20%?

Mostly what people are looking for from books such as this is a sure-fire way to reduce or control their weight. This section will provide that. But there is no magic wand.

At Cannons Sports Clubs we have been operating our special 20:30 Six-Week Weight Loss Programme since 1984 with 99% success rates – women lose eight to twelve pounds, men, a stone or more. Almost 2,000 have participated to date.

A similar 'inches off' programme has been added recently. We teach you to establish your own balanced eating programme so that the weight you lose will stay off. It is so simple once you know how and, like most things, the more you practise it, the easier it becomes.

The last section of this chapter shows how to best read the nutrient guide now compulsory in the grocery trade, and to spot the way these are sometimes displayed to mislead the casual buyer.

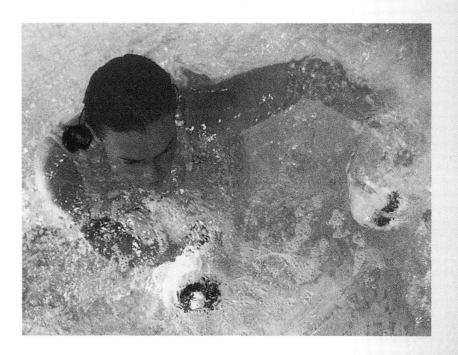

8 USE IT OR LOSE IT   *103*
The value of regular exercise

Some suggestions and recommendations, including water workouts and circuits which can be done anywhere

Once you know what you need to know about the body and its operation, about avoiding lifestyle diseases and about nutritional essentials and the merits of suntanning and weight control, then you are ready to explore the type of exercise which best suits you. Included is a simple twenty-minute circuit you can do at home, in the office or in a hotel room whilst travelling. You need never go a day without exercising.

We also explain how best to establish your aerobic threshold and how you can maximize the efficiency of your aerobic workouts with pulse rates.

9 KEEPING TRACK   *127*
Monitoring progress

Health and fitness tests

If you are eating correctly and exercising as well as you are able (or even if you are not), then you should be checking your progress regularly.

What chaos a rugby game would become, or any sort of sport for that matter, if no score was kept. How could a business check its progress, positive or negative, without keeping a tab via the trading accounts and balance sheets? Yet we rarely bother taking the same trouble with our own health or, if we do, we do it irregularly. We tell you how best to keep track of your physical improvement (or deterioration).

In our lifestyle questionnaire you can assess for yourself some of the important elements in your way of life and the risks you are taking living this way.

10 DOING IT SLOW AND EASY *141*

Some further advice on exercise and training, how any size, shape, age, or personality can benefit, and how to keep it interesting and challenging.

11 DIFFERENT WAYS OF   *147*
GOING ABOUT IT

There are many forms of exercise and recreation. Here are some you may not have thought about.

12 OUR WAY   *153*

Why should you follow our advice? Here is a short, final chapter about our philosophies and principles so that you know where our ideas and concepts are coming from.

PUBLISHER'S NOTE   *156*

REFERENCE LIST   *158*

FOREWORD

> **When I was young in Australia I swung upside down from trees**

Having run 5,000 metres against Ron Clarke on several occasions and matched him shoulder to shoulder in the home stretch, I can give other distance runners of our calibre the following tip for defeating him tactically: start ten minutes earlier. If you and he are both running on adjacent treadmills at Cannons, it can be done. A lot of things can be done for the human body at Cannons. Things have been done even for my body, which was probably the nearest to a total wreck that ever stumbled out of the locker room in baggy shorts and a too-tight T-shirt. I didn't get back my youth. I didn't get back the full splendour of that original V-shaped figure that stunned the beach so long ago. But I got my weight reasonably under control, regained the habit of exercise, and above all rediscovered the pleasure of a healthy sweat.

When I was young in Australia I swung upside down from trees, half-killed myself clown-diving at the baths, and rode my three-speed bike for 20 miles at a time through the storm-water channels of the Sydney suburbs. I burned energy as fast as I generated it. Then about 30 years went by when I burned no energy at all, with results that most of you can guess at and some of you know all too well. It is this latter group that I address now: we of a Certain Age, victims of Time's depredations, the invasion of the body-snatcher. The greatest danger we face, when we try to get our bodies back, is of overdoing it. The great virtue of a properly run gymnasium like Cannons is that we aren't allowed to. The staff are on the alert, making sure that no new member with one foot in the grave will try to pull it out so fast he sprains a thigh. The watchful dedication of these young guardians is eloquent testimony to how the health movement has calmed down from its initial wild enthusiasm and become part of the landscape instead of just a craze like the hula-hoop or Rubik's cube.

A craze was what it used to be. It all started with jogging. The so-called health editors of the Sunday newspapers filled pages with copy advising out-of-condition executives about where, when and how often to jog. One health editor was so impressed at his own easy breathing after a six-mile jog that he went off to do the same course again. Before he was half way around he wasn't breathing at all. The following week there was a new health editor. Like his predecessor he was really an out-of-condition executive himself. Jogging shattered many a calcified Achilles tendon before the general realization dawned that it had to be done under controlled conditions.

By the time that was grasped, the more trend-conscious out-of-condition executives had given up jogging and moved on to lifting weights. Men barely capable of lifting a double brandy were pounding themselves into the carpet lifting weights at home. They were the wrong weight. There was nothing wrong with the principle. There was just a lot wrong with the practise. People who had spent 30 years getting out of shape weren't going to get back into it in 30

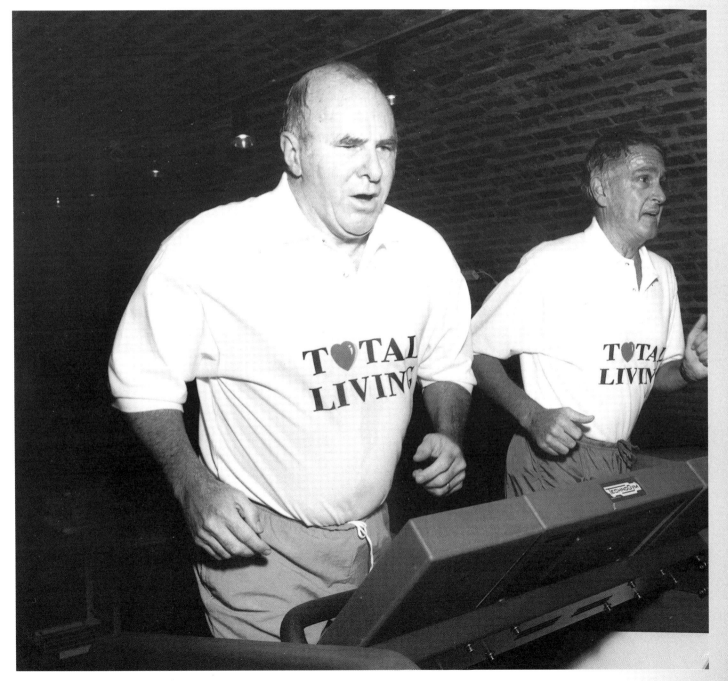

Matching Ron shoulder to shoulder.

FOREWORD

> **If I had my life over again I would spend most of it in the gym**

Anyone worried about the deceptive comfort of their swivel chair should seek to rekindle that old flame immediately.

minutes. Luckily the gymnasium movement arrived before they all ended up in traction.

The great majority of Cannons members, of course, are young executive types who have never been very far out of condition in the first place and consequently have little trouble either getting back into it or else simply maintaining an impeccable physique. I try not to hate them. Some of the women look very cute in leotards and I try not to ogle them, an activity reprehensible at my age, and no longer tolerated even amongst the young. But I can't help sneaking a sideways look at the aerobics classes. It must be fun to bounce around like that. Certainly it seems to induce an intense camaraderie. In the snack bar afterwards you can see the aerobics

experts describing their moments of glory to each other like fighter pilots after a dogfight. The après-sweat social facilities at Cannons improve after each rebuild of the premises. If I had my life over again I would spend most of it in the gym, staying in my magnificent original trim as I strode manfully between the Nautilus machines and the punching bags, writing my books at a cafeteria table with nothing to drink except a can of Dexter's, buffing up my immortality.

Life didn't work out that way. An old buffer has nothing left to buff up. But he can put the brakes on his decline, and feel hale again if not hearty. Like the other older senatorial figures who come to the gym I enjoy my solitude, the only hour in the day when nobody wants anything from me. You can see us in the sauna, each alone with his head in his hands, getting back in touch with the physical life, re-establishing the almost but not quite lost connection between the sound mind and sound body. There's something Roman about it. A thousand years from now, when they dig up the railway station, find a gymnasium underneath it, and decide that ours must have been an advanced civilization after all, they won't be far wrong. I can recommend without reservation that anyone worried about the deceptive comfort of his or her swivel chair should follow my lead and re-kindle that old flame immediately: don't let even a single decade go by.

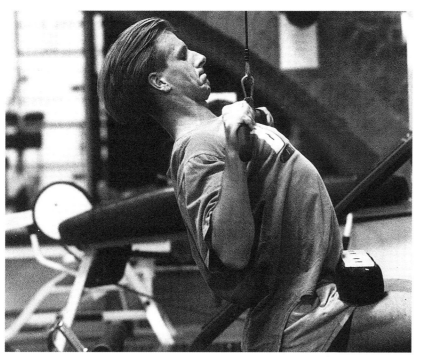

CLIVE JAMES, 1994

FOREWORD

Total living is a lifestyle to which we readily relate. People seem to think that we athletes, because we train so hard, have no time to enjoy the normal things. This is completely wrong.

In fact, training each day gives us an appreciation of how lucky we are, and how important it is for exercise to be part of a normal lifestyle. But it always remains just that, a part of our lives, no matter how dedicated we may be. Certainly there is no need for everyone to train with the intensity of an Olympic athlete, but even after retiring from international competition my routine would not be the same without some time devoted to exercising. I know I would not feel as well. And it is this feeling of well being and vitality, stimulated by the exercise and some nutritional care, that allows us to enjoy life so much. It is a chicken-and-egg situation really. The more regularly you exercise, the better you feel; the better you feel, the more regularly do you train.

When Sally and I first went to Cannons we were desperate to locate a gymnasium where we could augment our running training on a daily basis. Both of us had to earn our living from our office jobs, so we joined the throng of Cannons members who work out three or four times a week just to keep fit.

I suppose it was more critical than merely keeping fit to us, but nevertheless it was fun. The atmosphere at the club, the total lifestyle

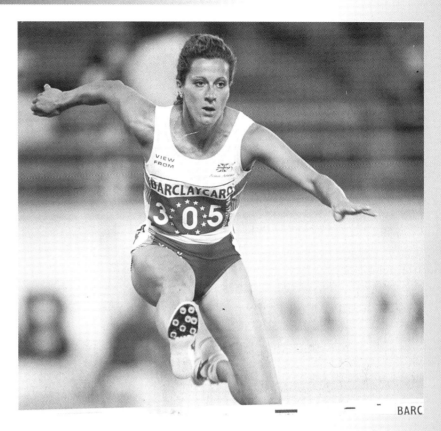

concept preached by Ron Clarke and his team, and the uniqueness and variety of their facilities, proved just perfect for us. I was lucky enough to attend three Olympics during my time there, and Sally two (and what an Olympics she had in Barcelona), but more importantly we share with all the Cannons people their approach to living, to taking some care about nutritional balancing, to fitting in easy but appropriate exercise sessions most days, and the sheer enjoyment that feeling of good health brings to us all.

KIM HAGGER AND SALLY GUNNELL, 1994

> *The more regularly you exercise, the better you feel*

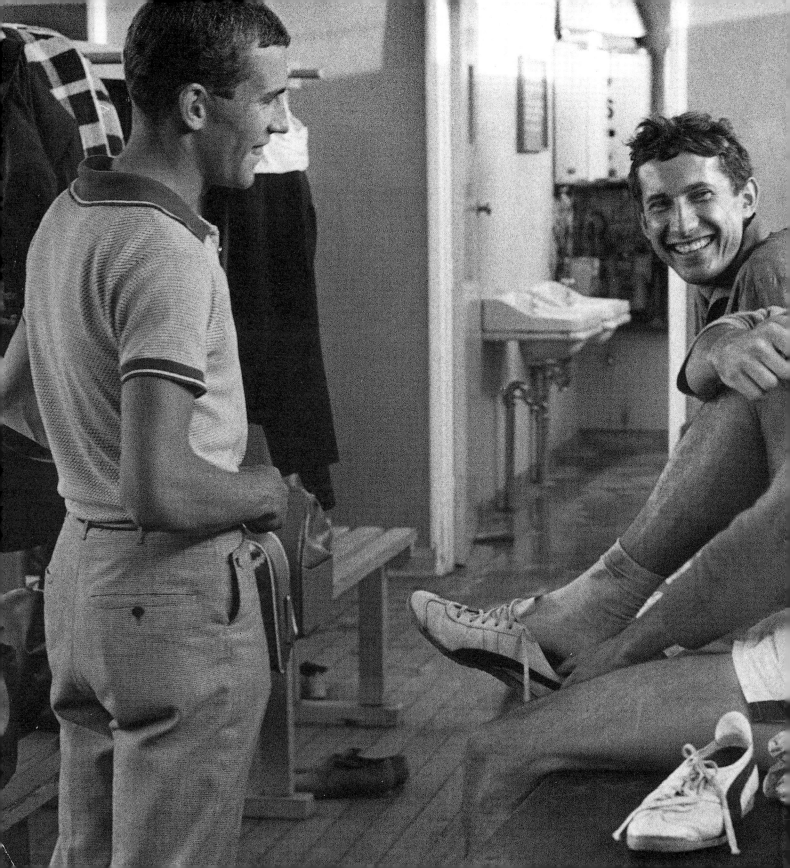

CHAPTER ONE

PATHWAY TO PARADISE

When I was just starting in the athletics business, a famous English distance runner, Gordon Pirie, gave me some good advice: *'One of the hardest things you will find about training is actually getting changed to go out.'*

And so it proved.

After returning home from the office late in the evening on cold, windy, wintry nights, I would find the comfort of playing with the children in front of the fire whilst Helen, my wife, prepared the evening meal in the adjoining kitchen, almost irresistible. If I had not been an international athlete, realized the necessity of consistent training, and remembered that early warning from Gordon, I am sure I would have succumbed to the warmth and comfort of home, and put off training for another day.

This comfort zone is even harder to break when it has become the habit of a lifetime.

That is why we have named this volume *Total Living.* Unless you take the initiative, and resolve that come what may an almost daily exercise routine will become a vital element in your new lifestyle, you will find it so easy to stay in the pipe-and-slipper comfort zone that has so many dangerous consequences. 'Why?' you may well ask. Because life is for living

'Why?' you may well ask. Because life is for living…

> *If your body and soul are properly toned, you can cope with a greater variety of 'the good life' than normal*

Very few have the genes to emulate the physique of a Linford Christie no matter how hard they work at it.

and without a total lifestyle which includes proper exercise and nutrition you are missing out badly.

The feel of a taut, tight body able to undertake any task with ease, a mind which can concentrate for six to ten hours at a time, a spirit which is always up, a temperament which copes equally well with the triumphs and disasters of daily business, not to mention family life, are all products of a simple, daily concern for a not-very-long workout and nutritional value in your meals.

For it is not just the regular exercise which is important, it is the whole gambit – what I like to call *Total Living* (just as those famous Dutch teams dubbed their new style of playing in the 1970s, *Total Football*).

Total living does **not** mean a routine of celery, exercise and off to bed at sundown. Rather, quite the opposite. If your body and soul are properly toned, you can cope with a greater variety of 'the good life' than normal. The fitter you are, the higher your reserves.

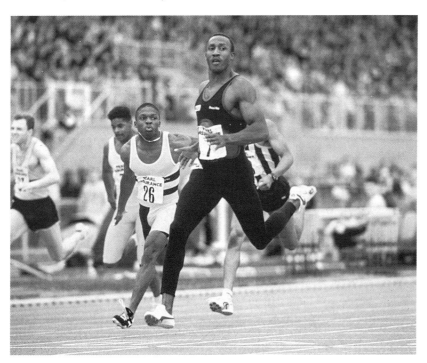

What we are talking about here, though, is not Olympic-level fitness, nor even the fitness levels of those dedicated souls you find in all sports who, whilst never reaching international or even national status, still train assiduously and regularly. They need no assistance from us.

What this book addresses is general health for the normal populace – who probably approach the subject by wondering *'How little do I need to do?'*, rather than the *'How much can I fit in today?'* of the genuinely athletically inclined.

Actually this is a fair question. Those who we wish to influence have not the time, the desire or the inclination to reach the dizzy heights of Total Fitness. But they do want to be healthy well into old age and this incorporates elements of:

♥ Luck (choosing your parents carefully)
♥ Nutrition (selecting sensible options)
♥ Exercise (making it time-efficient and interesting)
♥ Sensible monitoring (correct health screens and simple self-tests).

How lucky were you in the genetic stakes?

Luck is important in choosing the right parents because their genes are those which you carry and their body type, propensity to cancer and heart disease is a major factor in your own. Even the type of muscle fibre they pass on to you makes a substantial difference to your own lifestyle and to your likelihood of an early death. This does not mean that if, for example, both your parents died prematurely from heart disease, you are pre-ordained to follow them to an early grave. Nor, conversely, do long-living parents guarantee that you, too, will inherit their longevity.

But these are factors you must keep in mind when looking at ways to control your own life. In order to take charge all your possible weaknesses and strengths must be considered. This is why we ask you to examine your own lifestyle factors, and those of your parents, in our lifestyle questionnaire in chapter 9.

One other factor inherited from your antecedents, which is often ignored by physiologists when setting up appropriate exercise programmes, is your actual aerobic or anaerobic capacities.

Champion long-distance runners are both born and made. Nobody breaks a world record without first having inherited the right muscular chemistry and body type, and then having the determination to work on these gifts.

On the other hand, Linford Christie and his colleagues of similar muscular construction were born to be sprinters. They inherited the right physical make-up and most importantly a preponderence of so-called quick-twitching muscle fibres which allows them to propel their bodies that much faster than anyone else. Of course, they also have had to work their butts off to develop the necessary strength, technique and mental temperament which are also essential to become a champion sprinter.

Very few inherit such advantages, and a lot of those who do never have the good fortune to be exposed to the particular sport or activity for which they have the 'natural' ability.

And then there are those who have it and know it, but do not possess the relentless drive and determination to work on their talent in the way that the champions do.

Whatever, we are talking to you as a normal person, not one who has inherited great natural talent for anything in particular. Champion or not, you *will* have a natural tendency for *either* an aerobic (stamina) *or* a non-aerobic (quick-moving) ability.

Your muscles may not possess the quick-twitching capacity to match Lewis and Christie, nor the aerobic ability to circulate oxygen of a Coe, but they will have some characteristics you should identify. Any workouts you undertake should recognize these characteristics in the way the exercise programmes are put together.

For example, each of us should include some aerobic style workouts into our lifestyle on a regular basis as these are the means for improving the body's main functions, its heart, lungs and oxygen circulation (usually referred to as the cardio-respiratory system).

But those with aerobic genes will quickly come to terms with these workouts and will soon be able to comfortably cope with long runs, swims, walks or cycling – whichever choice they make.

Those with sprinter's genes, though, will find such workouts quite difficult no matter how long they persist. If you are one of this type, you should try what we call interval sessions in order to get the same effect, whilst indulging your own natural tendencies for fast movements. In an interval session, the distance is split into sections and you run (or walk, etc.) hard for up to two/three minutes, ease off and recover for two or three minutes, then repeat the effort. Ten of these efforts and you have gained the benefit of an aerobic session without having to endure the non-stop continuous effort which the pure stamina type usually prefers.

The effect, aerobically, is about the same but interval sessions appeal to those with a 'sprinter's' make-up, as do the longer continuous sessions to those with a natural stamina background.

More about this later. The point I wish to make here is that everybody is different and workouts can be varied to suit an individual's personal characteristics, and be equally effective.

You are what you eat

It was estimated recently that 70% of the adult population of the United Kingdom is overweight, and if that 70% reduced their weight by 10%, they would increase their chance of living an additional five years by 50%. The effect on the national economy would be enormous.

Everybody is different and workouts can be varied to suit an individual's personal characteristics, and be equally effective

Yet despite the fact that correct nutrition is so basic, it is still so misunderstood. Our aim is simply to get you to nutritionally balance your daily intake of food and drink as much as possible – so compensations can be made if, through circumstance or a particular liking, too much of one kind of food type has been consumed too often.

Fundamentally we recommend a 20:30:50 balance – 20% protein, 30% fat, 50% carbohydrate. Carbohydrate can go up to 55%, or protein to 25%, but the weekly fat content of your total food intake should never be more than 30%.

And, for those of you who need it, we show you some painless ways to lose 10% of your weight and keep it off. All is explained in chapter 7 on weight loss and nutrition.

No one expects you to starve, or to spend all your time analysing foodstuffs. But you should be able to devote a few minutes each day for a few weeks checking out the nutritional elements of your diet so that you can understand the concept of which food provides which nutritional gain, to what degree and how many calories it contains.

Exercise: it de-stresses as it invigorates

There are all types of exercise but, whatever you do, there should be one recurring theme – it should be challenging, yet easy; something that tests you, yet an activity you look forward to. If the very thought of exercise stresses you then forget it, you should just go out for a gentle walk. But remember you are placing your later years on to the wheel of fortune.

Frankly, I cannot imagine anyone with a dollop of spirit not being challenged by a spot of exercise. It is the best de-stressing agent I can think of. An aerobic class, swim or gym workout in the middle of the day gives you the chance to 're-oxygenize' your brain and body, recharge the little grey cells and generally tackle any problems with a renewed vigour.

Normally, the greatest obstacle to the average working person is time. How to organize the day to fit in a workout when an hour spent away from the desk, phone or business seems impossible.

In reality your own health is the most important asset you possess. If you are that valuable to the business that you cannot even be spared for 60 minutes or so, then all the more reason you should take steps to protect your health so you will be around for longer. If you get sick, somehow everybody copes, so it must be possible to fit in an hour or so before, during or after the working day. Frankly, no one is immortal, everybody is replaceable, and the excuse that you cannot spare 60 minutes away from the action is more a

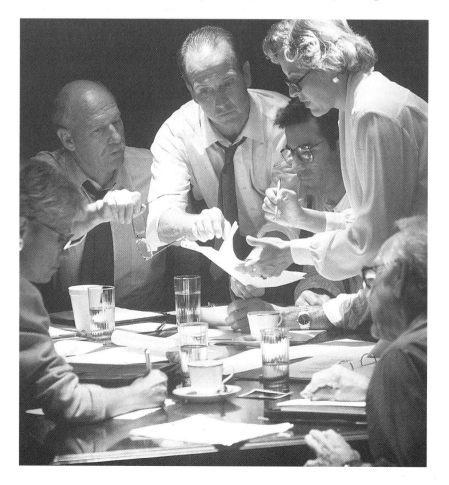

A spot of exercise is the best answer to stress there is; lunchtime workouts recharge the psyche and refresh the pyhsique.
Exercise de-stresses as it invigorates.

testimony to your inability to organize your day properly than proof of your indispensability. Why not sort out your day better and take some time away, for your own sake? You will be much the better for it.

Knowledge is everything

What most of us neglect to do about our health is to monitor it regularly. Those who train regularly feel there is no need to; those who do not are afraid to.

In this day and age, with the diagnostic and health screening techniques available, no one over the age of 35 should ignore regular testing so as to know his/her state of health at any time.

How could a business manage without periodic profit statements and balance sheets? Would anyone run a car without giving it a regular service and maintenance checks?

Yet most people regard regular health screenings as a waste of time; we feel well so we are well. We think we only need to see the doctor when we get sick. It is really stupid.

Everyone needs a regular check, at least yearly, of both fitness and health. In my opinion, employers should be made to provide these sorts of screenings for their staff each year as a part of their wage package. It is surely as important as providing staff rooms, toilet facilities and annual vacations.

We owe it to ourselves and to our families to look after ourselves in this way. Later, in chapter 9, we discuss the types of tests which you should insist upon having each year as these, too, vary according to your age, state of fitness and lifestyle.

We also look at getting old, at the young, and at some alternative lifestyles and activities which may attract your interest.

Start today

So there it is. In the pages which follow, we simply want to advise you how best you can look after yourself. Our aim has been to do it simply, succinctly and

attractively so you can have a good read and see exactly what you need do to improve your own lifestyle without losing one moment of enjoyment.

This is not meant to be a textbook. Our aim is to provide information on a 'need-to-know' basis. There is such a profusion of advice on health, so many people recommending this and that, confusing rather than enlightening their readers. We have tried to be different by being more direct and not expecting any great sacrifice from our readers whilst adapting to a healthier way of living.

We do feel we know what we are talking about when discussing health and fitness. At Cannons, we have assisted more than 20,000 Londoners in the eleven years we have been operating. Approximately 13,000 are still currently involved on a day-to-day basis as members. We succeed because we provide genuine, no-nonsense workout facilities for our members, with classes, equipment and teachers geared to provide serious, effective exercise. We do not specialize in the social events for members often revered by other clubs. Our people come, enjoy a workout, then go away happy after they have completed a worthwhile exercise session. They expect and get the best.

Be that as it may, in the end it really is up to you to shape the future you want to enjoy. We can show you how best to undertake a task, how to go about it, how to make it more interesting and varied, how to discover your weaknesses and ways to overcome these, *but we cannot make you do it.*

What we can do is repeat our plea: do not procrastinate, decide to get started, and then do something about it, today, by reading chapter 8 on exercise and undertaking your initial workout. It may be a 1,000-mile trip to get back to your prime, but every journey starts with one small step.

Those who train regularly feel there is no need to monitor their health; those who do not are afraid to

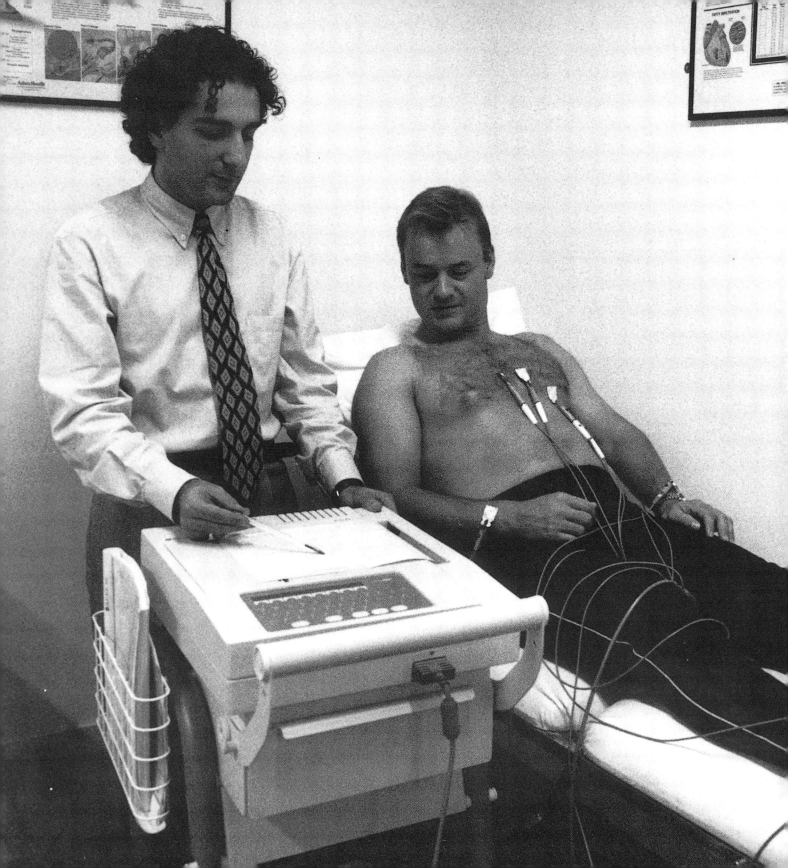

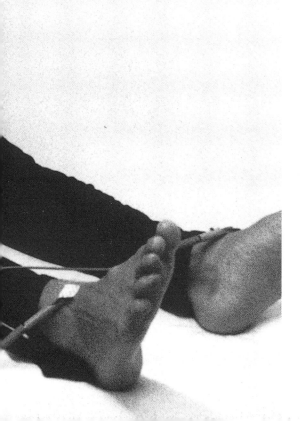

CHAPTER TWO

THE HEART OF THE MATTER

Before getting involved in any health improvement or health management programmes, the basic fundamental anatomy of the heart muscle, its functions and actions, and that of the body should be understood.

Most of our readers are probably very aware of these, but it never hurts to reiterate the basic facts: without a working knowledge of them, the very reason for exercise and sensible nutrition cannot be properly understood.

This chapter is particularly important to our female readers: although most women live in dread of their middle-aged husbands dropping dead from heart attacks, in actual fact they are just as much at risk themselves.

It has always been assumed that the high oestrogen levels in the female body protect women from heart attacks, but problems arise after the menopause which can occur as soon as the early forties.

Most women worry about cancer more than heart disease, but the fact is that three times as many of

Our risk of cardio-vascular disease is affected by many lifestyle factors

Figure 1

66

Three times as many women die of heart attacks than of ovarian, breast and uterine cancer combined

99

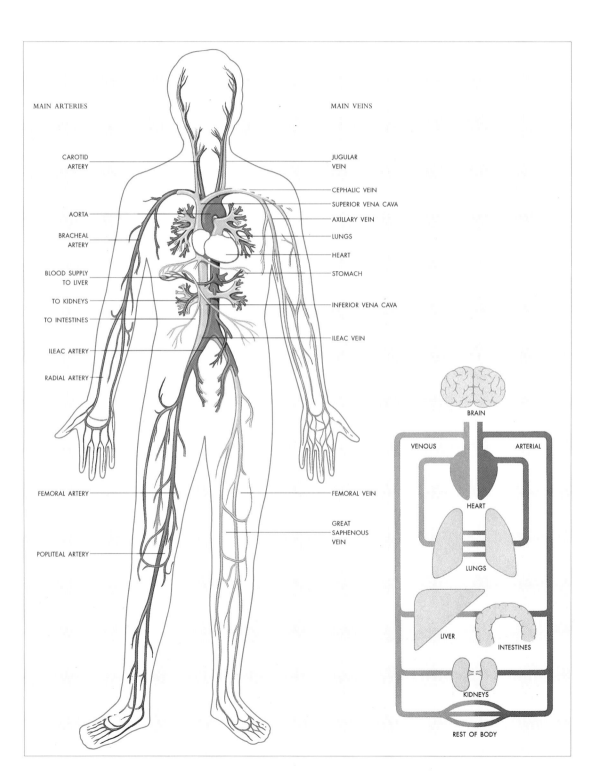

MAIN ARTERIES

CAROTID ARTERY
AORTA
BRACHEAL ARTERY
BLOOD SUPPLY TO LIVER
TO KIDNEYS
TO INTESTINES
ILEAC ARTERY
RADIAL ARTERY
FEMORAL ARTERY
POPLITEAL ARTERY

MAIN VEINS

JUGULAR VEIN
CEPHALIC VEIN
SUPERIOR VENA CAVA
AXILLARY VEIN
LUNGS
HEART
STOMACH
INFERIOR VENA CAVA
ILEAC VEIN
FEMORAL VEIN
GREAT SAPHENOUS VEIN

BRAIN
VENOUS
ARTERIAL
HEART
LUNGS
LIVER
INTESTINES
KIDNEYS
REST OF BODY

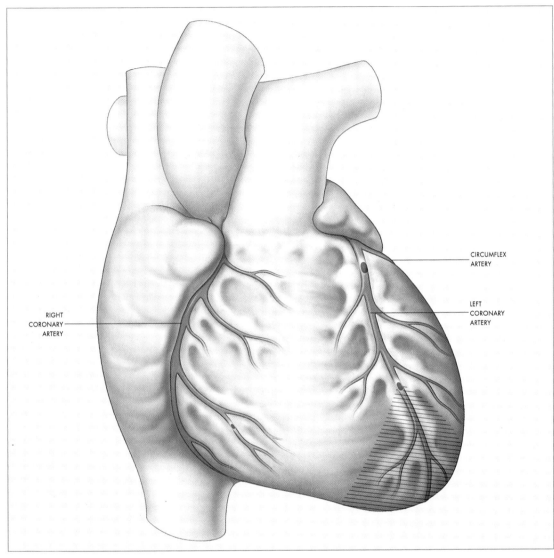

RIGHT
CORONARY
ARTERY

CIRCUMFLEX
ARTERY

LEFT
CORONARY
ARTERY

Figure 2

"

Although the heart is continually pumping blood through its internal chambers, it cannot use this blood to nourish its own muscle

"

them die of heart attacks than of ovarian, breast and uterine cancer combined.

Everybody therefore should take time out to read the following analysis from our consultant, Dr John Briffa. It is an easy-to-follow explanation of the various elements involved with heart function and disease.

Despite improvements in diagnosis and treatment, cardio-vascular disease (heart attacks and strokes) remains the leading cause of death in the industrialized world. According to the World Health Organization, of the 11 million deaths which occur each year in Western society, 25% are due to heart disease, and a further 13% are caused by strokes. The scale of the problem becomes even more alarming when you consider the body of evidence which suggests that many heart attacks and strokes could actually be prevented.

Our risk of cardio-vascular disease is affected by many lifestyle factors, such as what we eat and drink, whether we smoke or not, and how much exercise we take. Later, I will explain the relevance of these factors and describe how they may be modified to reduce our risk of heart attack and stroke.

However, in order to understand fully how best to protect ourselves from cardio-vascular illness, it is useful to have a working knowledge of the heart and circulation, and the internal process which gives rise to heart attacks and strokes called **atherosclerosis.**

The heart and circulation

The heart is a superb muscular pump, about the size of a fist, situated in the centre of the chest, between the lungs. Its function is to pump blood around the body, enabling essential substances such as oxygen and nutrients to be transported to every part of the body. Blood is pumped to various parts of the body in vessels called **arteries** and returns to the heart in **veins.**

The heart is divided into two. The right side pumps blood to the lungs where carbon dioxide is exchanged for oxygen. The oxygenated blood returns to the left side of the heart which then pumps the blood to every other part of the body. After oxygen is extracted from the blood by the tissues, the blood then returns to the right side of the heart to be pumped once more to the lungs (see figure 1).

At rest, the heart beats about 60–80 times each minute, which equates to about five litres of blood per minute. When demands are placed on the body, for instance when we exercise, the heart responds by beating more quickly and can actually pump up to about 25 litres of blood every minute at maximum output by increasing both the number of beats to around 200 and the actual volume of blood pumped with each stroke.

The coronary and cerebral arteries

Every organ in the body needs a blood supply and the heart is no exception. Although the heart is continually pumping blood through its internal chambers, it cannot use this blood to nourish its own muscle. The heart is supplied with blood from three **coronary arteries** which can be seen clearly on its surface (see figure 2).

The brain, too, has its own blood supply and receives this via the **cerebral arteries.**

What is cardio-vascular disease?

'Cardio-vascular disease' is a term used to describe both coronary heart disease (heart attacks and angina) and strokes. Although the symptoms of these two conditions are quite different, they are, in fact, the result of the same process. Both result from the clogging of arteries with a fat-like substance. This process produces a gradual narrowing of vessels and is called **atherosclerosis.**

Cardio-vascular disease
Atherosclerosis

The effects of atherosclerosis can take many years to come to light; scientific studies have shown that the

Figure 3

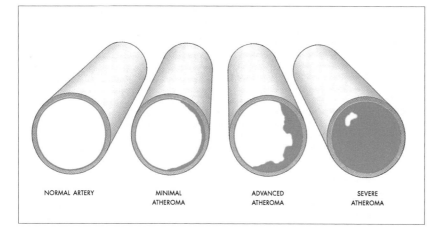

| NORMAL ARTERY | MINIMAL ATHEROMA | ADVANCED ATHEROMA | SEVERE ATHEROMA |

process may start in childhood or early adolescence. Over the years, more and more fatty substance is deposited in the arteries, all the time narrowing the vessel (see figure 3). If it becomes very blocked, then the tiniest blood clot (**thrombus**) is all that it may take to bring about a complete blockage of the artery.

What is a stroke?

A stroke occurs when a complete blockage of a cerebral artery causes part of the brain to be damaged or die. This may result in a variety of symptoms including speech problems, blindness and paralysis. The exact symptoms will depend on the precise part of the brain which is affected, and the extent of the damage. The medical term for stroke is **cerebro-vascular accident** or **CVA.**

What is a heart attack?

A heart attack results from a blockage in a coronary artery which causes some of the heart muscle to die. As with a stroke, the amount of heart muscle affected will depend on the precise site of the blockage. The larger the part of the heart which is damaged, the greater the risk of death. Death is also more common if a part of the heart is damaged which is essential to its function, such as an internal valve or part of the electrical circuitry which controls its contraction. Medical terms for heart attack include **myocardial infarction (MI)**, and **coronary infarction** (commonly known as a 'coronary').

Sometimes an individual may get symptoms of coronary heart disease before a full-blown heart attack. If the blood supply to the heart muscle is severely compromised, pain may be felt in the chest, particularly on exertion. This is called **angina pectoris** or, more simply, **angina**.

Prevention or cure?

Once someone has suffered a heart attack or stroke, the options for treatment are relatively limited. What is more, although some people may make remarkable recoveries after a stroke or heart attack, others can be left with severe, permanent disabilities.

By far the best approach is to **prevent** cardiovascular disease from occurring in the first place. To achieve this, we must do whatever we can to prevent or delay the process of atherosclerosis.

What causes atherosclerosis to develop?

Atherosclerosis does not usually result from a single, isolated cause. Many factors are known to increase the risk of atherosclerosis, and there is normally more than one factor at work in each individual.

The most important risk factors are:

♥ high blood cholesterol
♥ high blood pressure
♥ cigarette smoking
♥ overweight and obesity
♥ high blood sugar (diabetes)
♥ lack of physical exercise
♥ male sex
♥ increased age
♥ a family history of heart disease.

Although these factors are often quoted in relation to heart disease, they may each play a part in a stroke.

The greater the number of risk factors that apply to you, the greater your risk of heart disease. Three factors (sex, age and family history) are unfortunately beyond our control. However, we do have the ability to influence the remainder, and scientific studies are proving just how effective modifying these risk factors can be. For instance, if a 40-year-old man reduces his cholesterol by about 10%, his risk of heart disease may be effectively **halved** in the long term.

If a 40-year-old man reduces his cholesterol by about 10%, his risk of heart disease is effectively halved

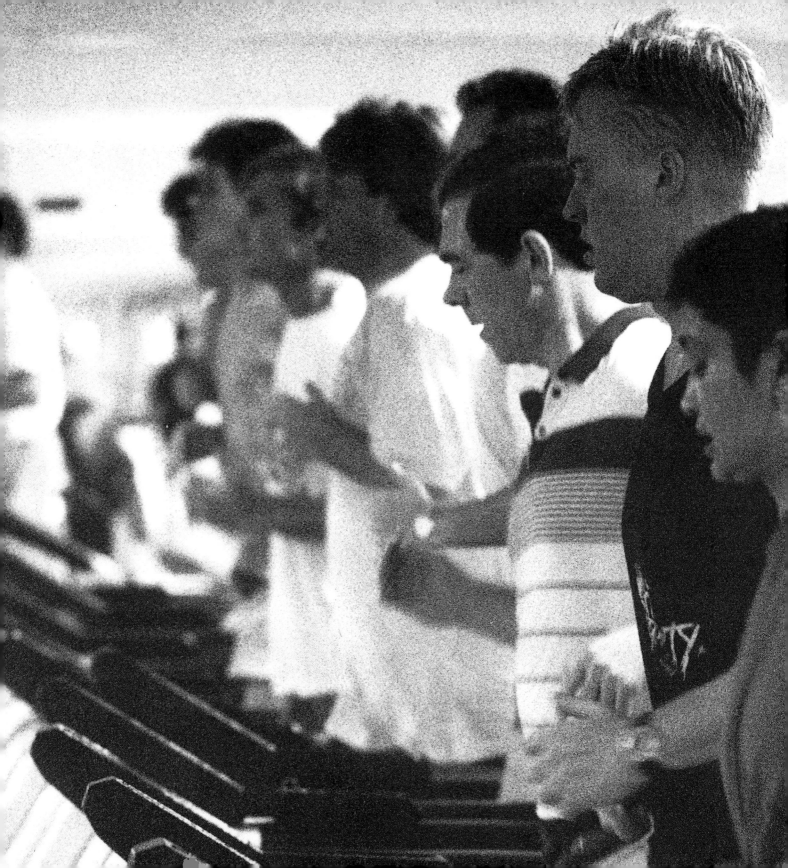

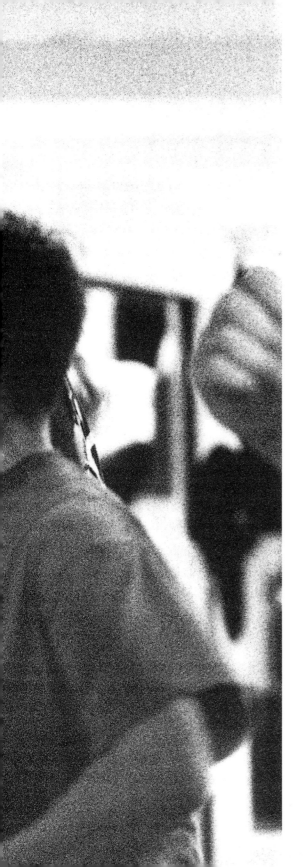

CHAPTER THREE

STAYING ALIVE

This chapter takes an in-depth look at the major controllable risk factors for cardio-vascular disease. These are: blood cholesterol, blood pressure, smoking, body weight, blood sugar and physical exercise.

The mechanisms which influence each of these risk factors will be discussed, and practical advice will be given on how we can reduce our risk of cardio-vascular disease using simple lifestyle changes.

Cholesterol and Cardio-vascular Disease

Many experts regard high blood cholesterol as one of the most important risk factors for developing heart disease. Anyone can develop a high cholesterol level regardless of age, sex and race. Because there are no obvious warning signs, we cannot be sure whether or not we have a problem unless our cholesterol level is measured. If it is found to be high, changing our diet can be very effective in bringing cholesterol down, and reducing our risk of heart disease.

What is cholesterol?

Cholesterol is a type of fat and comes in a variety of different forms. Although too much is a bad thing,

> *Blood cholesterol – one of the most important risk factors for developing heart disease*

some cholesterol is important in the manufacture of cell walls, hormones and bile in the gut.

Where does cholesterol come from?

Cholesterol in the body either comes from the diet, or is manufactured by the liver. It is the dietary component which is important, because this is the part we can influence by reducing our intake of fat, and even relatively small changes in blood cholesterol may have significant benefit.

When fat is eaten, it is broken down (digested) in the gut and then passed into the bloodstream. Fat does not dissolve in blood, and so it needs to be 'packaged' before it can be transported around the body. Fat particles are wrapped in protein to make tiny parcels which are called **lipoproteins** for transportation.

What function do lipoproteins have?

There are two basic types of lipoprotein: **high density** lipoproteins (HDLs) and **low density** lipoproteins (LDLs). LDL has the function of transporting fat around the body to deposit it at various sites, including the coronary and cerebral arteries. LDL therefore plays a part in the development of atherosclerosis and is sometimes referred to as 'bad cholesterol'.

HDL, on the other hand, can take fat and help remove it from the body through the production of bile in the gut. HDL seems to have the opposite effect to LDL and is therefore sometimes referred to as 'good cholesterol'.

What is the relevance of the cholesterol level?

Generally speaking, the more cholesterol you have circulating in your bloodstream, the more likely you are to suffer from atherosclerosis and heart disease. Blood cholesterol is measured in units known as millimoles per litre of blood (mmol/l).

Some cholesterol is important in the manufacture of cell walls, hormones and bile in the gut

The following table is a guide to the risk associated with cholesterol concentration.

- ♥ **Blood cholesterol 5.2mmol/l or less:**
  This is a desirable cholesterol level.
- ♥ **Blood cholesterol between 5.2 and 6.5mmol/l:**
  Blood cholesterol is moderately raised. This level of cholesterol is associated with an increased risk of heart disease.
- ♥ **Blood cholesterol more than 6.5mmol/l:**
  Blood cholesterol is significantly raised. Risk of heart disease at this level may be marked.

Although the level of total cholesterol in the blood is important, it is not the whole story. If the level of total cholesterol is raised, then the relative proportions of LDL and HDL are of prime importance.

How are the relative amounts of LDL and HDL important?

If total cholesterol is raised, it is essential to know the ratio of total cholesterol (TC) to HDL. As TC is mainly LDL ('bad cholesterol'), and HDL is 'good cholesterol', the more TC there is to HDL, the greater the risk. It is generally accepted that a TC:HDL ratio of 5 or more adds significantly to the risk of a raised total cholesterol..

What are triglycerides?

Should you ever have your cholesterol assessed by laboratory analysis, your triglyceride level may be measured also. Triglycerides are fats, but do not have the same structure as cholesterol. Like cholesterol, however, it seems that triglycerides do play a part in heart disease, although their role is unclear. The studies undertaken in Germany and Finland showed that men with a TC:HDL ratio of more than five and a triglyceride level of more than 2.3mmol/l, had sixteen to twenty times the risk of heart disease of men with low TC:HDL ratios and triglyceride levels under 2.3mmol/l.

Are the risk factors for men and women different?

Most of the information on risk factors for heart disease has come from studying groups of men. The question is, can we apply the same data to women? Recent studies suggest not.

Swedish research has found triglyceride levels to be of greater significance than cholesterol in women. A recent study showed that women with the highest levels of triglycerides had seven times the risk of dying from heart attack compared to the women with the lowest triglyceride levels.

Reducing cholesterol levels in the blood

Blood cholesterol levels can be reduced by limiting the amount of fat in our diet. However, not all dietary fats are the same: some are associated with heart disease, while others seem to protect against it. In order to make the healthiest dietary choices, we must know something about the different types of fats, and the foods in which they are found.

What are the different types of fat?

Fats can be broadly divided into three categories: saturated, mono-unsaturated and poly-unsaturated. Diets high in saturated fats are strongly linked with heart disease. Saturated fats are mainly to be found in animal produce such as meat, eggs, whole milk, cheese, cream and butter. Foods such as chocolate, cakes and biscuits are also high in saturated fat as are many other processed foods.

Diets high in mono-unsaturated and poly-unsaturated fats do not have the same strong links with heart disease as saturated fats, and many scientists believe they can actually help protect us from this condition. Mono-unsaturated fats include olive oil, almond oil and avocado oil. Poly-unsaturated fat is found in fish, and is the main constituent of various vegetable oils: sunflower, safflower, sesame and grape-seed oil, for example.

Eating for a lower cholesterol level

In general we eat too much fat. Reducing cholesterol levels can be achieved by limiting overall fat intake, while at the same time eating more unsaturated fats compared to the saturated variety.

These guidelines will help you to achieve this:

♥ **Eat lean meat** and cut off any visible fat.
♥ **Eat poultry rather than red meats** wherever possible. Poultry fat is mainly in the skin, so be sure to remove it.
♥ Better still, **eat more fish**. Oily fish such as herring, mackerel, tuna and trout are high in unsaturated fats which may well protect against heart disease.
♥ **Moderate your consumption of eggs and dairy products** such as cheese, whole milk, cream and butter. Choose low-fat varieties wherever possible, e.g. semi-skimmed or skimmed milk, cottage cheese, low-fat yoghurts. It is now thought that margarines have no significant health value over butter; it is best to limit the use of both margarine and butter.
♥ **Moderate your consumption of chocolate, cakes and biscuits.** Not only are these foods high in saturated fat, they also contain little in the way of fibre, vitamins or minerals.
♥ As much as possible, **avoid frying food.** Grilling, baking, steaming, boiling and microwaving are all much healthier ways you can use to prepare food.
♥ When you do use oil in cooking, make sure it is a **vegetable oil**. Extra virgin olive oil is a good choice and is thought to be one of the

In order to make the healthiest dietary choices, we must know something about the types of fats, and the foods in which they are found

There is growing evidence that high blood pressure can be effectively managed by modifying lifestyle factors

reasons Mediterranean races have a low incidence of heart disease.

Oat bran to reduce blood cholesterol

Since the 1960s, some scientists have believed that oat bran may have cholesterol-lowering properties. A study conducted in 1992 at the University of Minnesota, which analysed available data about oat bran, concluded that it can be valuable in reducing blood cholesterol levels. The results showed that oat bran, taken regularly, can decrease blood cholesterol by up to 5% (about 0.3mmol/l) and that this decrease is over and above that which could be achieved by a low cholesterol diet alone. The amount of oat bran needed to achieve this is about five grams per day.

Blood Pressure and Cardio-vascular Disease

High blood pressure is an important risk factor for

Does reducing your cholesterol actually reduce your risk of heart disease?

The answer to this question is an emphatic 'yes'. A recent analysis of data from half a million men published in the British Medical Journal in February 1994 showed that the risk of heart disease at all ages could be dramatically reduced by lowering blood cholesterol.

Not surprisingly, however, most benefit is to be had if changes are made earlier, rather than later in life.

The study showed the following overall reductions in the incidence of heart disease which may be achieved by a reduction in blood cholesterol of 0.6mmol/l (about 10%), achieved by moderate dietary change.

The study also showed that the full reduction in risk is achieved after five years.

The message is clear: reducing our blood

Decrease in incidence of heart disease linked to age

cholesterol concentration by cutting down on our consumption of fats can significantly reduce our chances of developing heart disease in the future. What is more, the sooner we start, the greater the benefit we enjoy.

heart disease, and is probably **the most important risk factor for stroke**. About one in ten people suffer from high blood pressure, and there are usually no associated symptoms. **Many people with high blood pressure are unaware that they have a problem**. This makes regular blood pressure checks an important part of any health programme.

There is growing evidence that high blood pressure can be effectively managed by modifying lifestyle factors. This section describes the factors which may contribute to high blood pressure, and sets out the simple measures which we can take to reduce it.

What does blood pressure measure?

The heart beats rhythmically to pump blood around the body. After the heart contracts to force blood out of the heart, it rests for a moment while it fills with blood before pumping again. The contraction phase of the cycle is known as **systole**, while the resting phase is called **diastole**.

The pressure of blood in our arteries is not constant, but varies according to the state of contraction of the heart. The measurement of blood pressure is presented as two figures. The upper figure is the pressure in the arteries when the heart is contracting and is known as the **systolic pressure**. The lower figure is the pressure in the system when the heart is in a relaxed state between beats and is termed the **diastolic pressure**. These two figures are normally expressed in millimetres of mercury (mmHg), with one figure on top of the other, e.g. 120/80mmHg.

What is high blood pressure (hypertension)?

Our blood pressure can go up and down according to what we are doing. For example, during exercise it is likely to be higher than at rest. But this is not what we mean by high blood pressure – it is flexible and quickly returns to normal levels once the exercise ceases. The hypertension type of high blood pressure

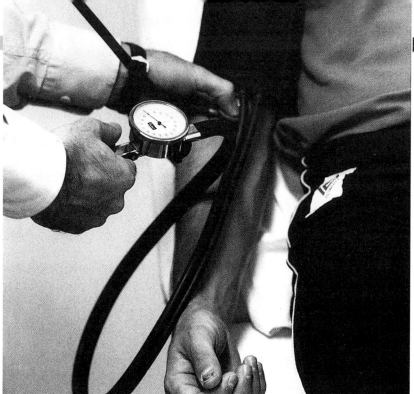

In expert hands, taking blood pressure is a quick, simple and painless procedure.

occurs when there is a chronic, lasting picture of high blood pressure and is almost always associated with atherosclerosis.

Because of the factor of variability, high blood pressure is very rarely diagnosed on the basis of one measurement. In order to be sure that an individual really does have high blood pressure, it is usually necessary to take several blood pressure readings, spread over several weeks or months.

There is no precise cut-off point between normal blood pressure and hypertension. Doctors find it hard to agree on parameters for this condition.

The following classification for blood pressure can be used as a guide:

Blood Pressure Classification

♥ **Normal**   A blood pressure of 140/90 or lower.

♥ **Borderline**   A systolic pressure of more than 140 but less than 160. A diastolic pressure of more than 90 but less than 100.

♥ **High blood pressure**   A systolic pressure of 160 or more. A diastolic pressure of 100 or more.

Some people ask which is more important, the systolic or diastolic pressure? There is no consensus at this time on which is more important, though there is little doubt that both are important in their own way.

What are the symptoms of hypertension?

Contrary to popular opinion, hypertension usually has no associated symptoms. Occasionally hypertension causes headaches, but this is the exception. Most people who suffer headaches have normal blood pressure.

What causes high blood pressure?

Like cardio-vascular disease, high blood pressure is not normally the result of one specific factor.

Six major risk factors for high blood pressure are:

♥ High salt consumption
♥ High alcohol consumption
♥ High stress levels
♥ Overweight and obesity
♥ Smoking
♥ Lack of physical exercise.

Three of these factors (obesity, smoking and lack of exercise) have already been mentioned as important risk factors for cardio-vascular disease in general. These factors will be discussed later in this chapter. The other three factors (salt, alcohol and stress) are discussed below.

Salt and high blood pressure

For many years a debate has raged in scientific circles about the relative importance of salt in high blood pressure. The latest evidence would suggest that salt is, indeed, an important factor in this condition.

A recent study undertaken at St Bartholomew's Hospital in London, has found that it is possible to predict the influence of salt on blood pressure quite

To be sure that an individual does have high blood pressure, it is usually necessary to take several blood pressure readings, spread over several weeks or months

accurately, and that the effect is greater than had been previously supposed.

The main findings of this study were:

- ♥ If everyone cut their salt intake by 30%, there would be a 22% fall in deaths from stroke and the number of people requiring treatment for hypertension would be halved.
- ♥ If we cut salt intake by 60%, then stroke deaths would fall by 39% and the number of people requiring medication for hypertension would be cut by a massive 80%.
- ♥ A salt reduction of 30% would result in a reduction in deaths from coronary heart disease of 16%, while a reduction of 30% in deaths would come about as a result of a 60% cut in salt intake.
- ♥ The older you are, and the higher your blood pressure, the greater the fall you can expect by reducing your salt intake.
- ♥ It takes more than five weeks of salt restriction to see the full change in blood pressure.

How can I achieve the reductions in salt consumption suggested?

Salt in the diet basically comes in two forms: the salt we add during cooking or at the table, and the salt already present in food (usually processed food). To effect the reductions suggested above is a relatively simple matter:

- ♥ **To reduce salt consumption by 30%:**
  Don't add salt during cooking or at the table.
- ♥ **To reduce salt consumption by 60%:**
  Don't add salt during cooking or at the table or eat processed foods with salt added.

The following is a list of food types which are likely to have significant amounts of salt already added to them. Wherever possible, read the ingredient labels on foods to find out how much salt they contain.

- ♥ Bacon, ham, salt beef, sausages, burgers, pies and canned meat
- ♥ Fish fingers, shell fish, smoked and tinned fish
- ♥ Instant meals, particularly those in pots
- ♥ Some breakfast cereals including high-fibre cereals described as 'healthy'
- ♥ Tinned and packet soups and sauces
- ♥ Stock cubes and yeast extracts
- ♥ Butter (except unsalted) and margarine
- ♥ Crisps, salted nuts and other snacks.

Alcohol consumption and high blood pressure

Salt restriction is not the only dietary measure that we should undertake to help control our blood pressure; it is sensible to reduce alcohol consumption too.

Researchers at the University of Western Australia, headed by Professor Laurie Beilin, have found that alcohol is highly potent at raising blood pressure, especially in binge drinkers. Reducing alcohol intake to one standard drink per day and avoiding heavy bouts has been shown to lower blood pressure considerably. Weight loss appears to add to this effect too.

In this study a group of overweight men enjoyed a reduction in blood pressure of ten points after shedding 10kg in five months and reducing their drinking by 80% on average.

Alcohol, heart disease and mortality

Most of us are familiar with the idea that a moderate amount of alcohol may be good for us. More and more research is being done which tends to support this idea. Many studies have shown that male and female abstainers have a higher risk of developing heart disease than people who consume moderate amounts. The precise explanation for this remains unclear, although it is now known that alcohol raises HDL levels (by about 15% on average), and reduces the tendency of the blood to clot. Too much alcohol, however, can actually increase the clotting tendency of blood.

Moderate alcohol consumption is also associated with reduced death rate from all causes. If a graph is plotted of death against alcohol consumption, the result is a J-shaped curve. On the left are the tee-totallers who are at increased risk, while on the right, those who consume excessive amounts of alcohol are at high risk too. However, the curve has a wide base, and it takes quite a lot of alcohol before a drinker's risk of mortality equals that of the teetotaller.

Alcohol consumption is usually measured in units of alcohol per week, where a unit of alcohol is equivalent to one glass of wine, a single measure of spirit, or half a pint (about 30cl) of beer. Sir Richard Doll of the Radcliffe Royal Infirmary in Oxford, England, calculated, in a study of male doctors, that the point at which a drinker's risk of mortality is the same as that of a teetotaller is at an alcohol intake of 42 units per week.

Moderate alcohol consumption is associated with a reduced risk of stroke, and elderly moderate drinkers retain better brain function and have denser bones than abstainers or heavy drinkers. Although the benefits of alcohol in moderation are not in doubt, scientists have not been able to agree on what actually constitutes the 'safest level'. A recent Danish study put the level at one to six units per week. One by the American Cancer Society puts the optimum drinking level at 10.5 units per week. John Duffy of the Alcohol Research Group at Edinburgh University has calculated the risk of death from any cause to be minimized at 26–30 units of alcohol per week.

We must not forget the terrible consequences of excessive alcohol consumption, however, from high blood pressure and cirrhosis of the liver and cancer, to the domestic, economic and social consequences of alcoholism. Fortunately, these effects result only from either very high levels of alcohol consumption, or from binge drinking.

In the light of such evidence, what conclusions can be drawn? One fact which appears not to be in dispute is that moderate alcohol consumption can help protect against heart disease and reduce overall mortality rates. However, the optimum level of drinking probably varies from individual to individual. Overall, the message seems to be: drink sensibly, spread your drinking over the whole week, and avoid getting drunk.

Stress and high blood pressure

Many people believe that because hypertension has the word 'tension' in it, then stress must have something to do with it. In fact, the role of stress in high blood pressure is far from clear.

One major reason why there is little firm evidence implicating stress in hypertension, is that it is actually very difficult to measure the psyche. It is hard enough evaluating, say, salt intake, and even more so the state of the mind. However, studies published in the *Journal of the American Medical Association* in 1993 have perhaps thrown a little more light on the question of the link between stress and high blood pressure.

The study followed over 1,100 middle-aged and elderly men and women over a period of twenty years. At the start of the study they had normal blood pressure, and the researchers wanted to see what role tension might have played in those who went on to develop hypertension.

They showed that stress only had a significant effect in middle-aged men with very high levels of anxiety. They had twice the chance of developing hypertension compared to men with low levels of anxiety.

Interestingly, none of the psychological states measured seemed to influence women's chances of high blood pressure. For women, it appears the most important factors in predicting risk of hypertension were initial weight, and whether they had a tendency to develop diabetes in later life. Although this study has not settled the continuing debate about stress and high blood pressure, it may be useful in pointing towards

The role of stress in high blood pressure is far from clear

highly stressed middle-aged men as a group which would benefit most from stress reduction.

Good and bad stress

Although stress has a somewhat negative association these days, it is not invariably a bad thing. Some of our most fulfilling moments can come in times of great stress. Psychologists have for some time been working on what it is about stress that determines its effect. The conclusions they draw may have important implications for the future of stress management.

Studies conducted over recent decades have shown that animals kept in environments which they cannot control become morose, develop ulcers, and may even die as a result. 'Learned helplessness' is the term used to describe such a situation, and it seems that stress, anxiety and depression are likely outcomes.

Control seems to be the important factor in stress

Scientists like Dr Martin Seligman from Cornell University in the US claim that the underlying factor for these effects, in animal and humans, is **uncontrollability**. Even if this lack of control is perceived and not real, Dr Seligman maintains that stress will result, often accompanied by other debilitating effects. It is likely that it is just this factor which explains why people who work in apparently stressful situations, such as the police and politicians, do not seem to suffer the effects of stress, while others appear to suffer in what *seem to be less stressful circumstances*.

In a review of means of coping with stress and helplessness, Dr Seligman claims that perceived control is largely a psychological factor (we are in control if we think we are in control), and as a result, coping mechanisms may be learnt which work by changing thought patterns.

Dr Seligman promotes a sense of control by changing thought patterns to believe that depressive or uncontrollable situations are not personal, permanent

and pervasive. Other analysts claim that relaxation training allows time and the framework for re-establishing control to manage stress.

However it is achieved, much of the psychological research on stress management is now looking towards a means of re-establishing control in individuals.

High blood pressure is a potent risk factor for cardio-vascular disease, particularly stroke. However, a reduction in salt intake, sensible drinking and effective stress control may each be effective in achieving natural blood pressure reduction.

Other means which may be used to control blood pressure include stopping smoking, losing weight and taking regular exercise. The remainder of this chapter deals with the effect of these, and also one other factor (diabetes) on our risk from cardio-vascular disease.

Cigarette Smoking and Cardio-vascular Disease

Cigarette smoking represents the biggest contributor to premature death in the Western world. It is not only associated with an increased risk of heart disease and stroke, but also with many forms of cancer and chronic lung conditions. If you smoke, the most important single contribution you can make to your future health and well-being is to stop.

Trends in cigarette smoking

The proportion of smokers in most industrialized nations is dropping by about 1% per year. Smoking seems to be declining in the higher socio-economic groups, while there has been relatively little change in the lower social classes. In some sectors, smoking even appears to be on the increase. For instance, in Britain, more and more young women are taking up smoking – possibly because smoking is thought to dull the appetite and therefore help as a slimming aid.

How does smoking cause disease?

Chemical analysis of tobacco smoke reveals almost 4,000 chemical compounds, more than 50 of which are known to be cancer-causing agents (carcinogens).

Nicotine itself can damage the heart, and the inhalation of cigarette smoke causes an increase in heart rate, an increase in blood pressure, and undesirable changes in the composition of the blood. Tobacco smoke also contains a gas called carbon monoxide, which is also present in high concentration in car exhaust fumes. The blood carries carbon monoxide in preference to oxygen, so smoking reduces the normal oxygen-carrying capacity of blood considerably. There is even some evidence to suggest that carbon monoxide in blood accelerates the formation of atherosclerosis.

What are the risks of cigarette smoking?

It is estimated that each cigarette smoked shortens the smoker's life by five and a half minutes. Smoking twenty cigarettes a day increases the risk of heart disease by **300%**, and the risk of lung cancer goes up by a massive **500%**. Ninety per cent of all lung cancers and chronic lung diseases such as emphysema and chronic bronchitis are caused by smoking.

Smoking not only increases *your* risk of disease, but also the risk to those around you. It has recently been estimated that, in the US alone, 53,000 non-smokers die each year from diseases caused by passive smoking. A recent study published in the *British Medical Journal* cited passive smoking as an important factor in a large number of chest infections and cases of asthma.

The effect of passive smoking on our children should not be forgotten. Research conducted at the University of Western Australia has shown that the younger the children are, the greater the dose of tobacco smoke they are likely to receive through passive smoking, and the more prone they are to suffer from respiratory problems such as asthma.

So why do we do it?

Well, quite simply, smoking is addictive. Smoking for most people starts as a purely recreational habit. We smoke our first cigarettes either through curiosity, or perhaps through peer pressure. At the outset, we go several days, weeks or months between cigarettes. Gradually, the time between each cigarette becomes shorter and shorter, and we can soon find ourselves smoking every day. Pretty soon cigarettes are no longer a small indulgence, but a necessity.

To understand how we can tackle the task of stopping smoking, we must first understand the nature of cigarette addiction itself. Cigarettes, like most other addictions, have two components to their addictive quality:

♥ physical addiction
♥ psychological addiction.

Physical addiction

When an addicted smoker stops smoking, he or she may experience a variety of withdrawal symptoms, which include:

♥ anxiety
♥ irritability
♥ coffee craving
♥ food cravings
♥ headache.

Nicotine withdrawal is at the root of these symptoms. The body has become accustomed to having regular doses of nicotine, and when the nicotine is no longer available, the body's internal balance is thrown out of line. All drugs which are physically addictive do this to some extent. Nicotine withdrawal is like a mild form of the withdrawal state known as 'cold turkey' associated with heroin use.

The physical element of nicotine addiction is actually relatively small. The symptoms are generally mild, and last anything from a few days to a few weeks. However, the ease with which we deal with these withdrawal symptoms depends largely on our degree of psychological addiction.

" Smoking twenty cigarettes a day increases the risk of heart disease by 300%, and the risk of lung cancer goes up by a massive 500% "

Gradually, the time between each cigarette becomes shorter and shorter – cigarettes are no longer a small indulgence, but a necessity

Psychological addiction

The psychological component of nicotine addiction is often ignored. But you must recognize this element of addiction if you are to deal with it successfully.

The majority of people who are planning to quit smoking convince themselves that it is going to be hell. They may have tried unsuccessfully to quit several times before, or may have heard stories from friends about how they tried and failed to stop smoking.

Individuals attempting to kick the habit tend to focus on the negative aspects of stopping smoking. They cannot imagine what life may be like without cigarettes. What are they going to do with their hands, and what are they going to do after meals, and after sex? Stopping smoking for these people is always going to be an uphill struggle because they are always going to believe they are missing out on something. It is these people who suffer regular pangs for cigarettes, long after the physical addiction has gone.

Dealing with psychological addiction

A positive mental attitude is essential. Instead of focusing on what we believe we will miss about smoking, we must concentrate on the many positive reasons there are for stopping. These are obviously a personal matter, but motives may include:

♥ to enjoy better health
♥ the better health of those around you, including your family
♥ not having to plan your life around your smoking habit
♥ not having to rush your meals just so that you can have a cigarette
♥ not having to sneak out of your non-smoking office for clandestine cigarettes

♥ more disposable income
♥ fresher smelling breath and clothes
♥ a real sense of achievement.

When you come to stop smoking, you must remind yourself of these reasons throughout the day, especially if you are tempted to smoke. Always remember what a huge favour you are doing yourself by quitting, and that you have nothing to lose, and everything to gain.

Dealing with physical addiction

Over the last few years there has been considerable interest in commercially available nicotine treatments which are aimed at lessening or eliminating the physical component of nicotine addiction. Currently, three such treatments exist. These are:

♥ Nicotine chewing gum (nicotine absorbed through the mouth)
♥ Nicotine patch (nicotine absorbed through the skin)
♥ Nicotine inhaler (nicotine absorbed through the lungs).

A group at St Bartholomew's Hospital in London recently reviewed the data from nearly 30 studies of the effectiveness of nicotine patches and chewing gum in around 11,000 people. The group made the following conclusions:

♥ Nicotine treatment should only be used in people who demonstrate a significant dependence on cigarettes.
(Factors which may suggest dependence include smoking more than ten cigarettes per day, smoking soon after getting out of bed, being tempted to smoke even in places where it is forbidden, and smoking when ill in bed.)
♥ The patch should be used in preference to the gum, except in highly dependent smokers, as it is better tolerated.
♥ In highly dependent smokers, the higher-strength chewing gum (4mg) is the treatment of choice.
♥ The gum and patches should be used for three months in carefully declining doses.

♥ The new nicotine inhalers should be used with care as they may give rise to addictive problems of their own and may cause irritation.

Please note that nicotine replacement is generally not recommended for people with heart disease or women who are pregnant. And do consult your doctor before commencing any such programme.

Choosing the day
It is very easy to find reasons why today is not a good day to stop smoking. Although the day should not be delayed indefinitely, it is probably a good idea to plan a couple of weeks in advance. Use this time to prepare yourself mentally. Keep going over in your mind the many positive reasons you have for stopping.

The day you stop smoking should not be viewed with fear or trepidation; it is a reason to celebrate. Smoke your last cigarette and tell yourself truthfully that it really will be your last. From this point on you are not giving up, you are a 'non-smoker'.

Staying stopped
Gradually, your body will eliminate nicotine from the system. While this is happening you may experience some of the symptoms mentioned above. Be prepared for these, but remember, as long as you keep a positive attitude, the effects will be manageable.

Over a few days or weeks you will notice these symptoms of withdrawal less and less. Remember to reward yourself each day. Think of what a great thing you are doing and savour the sense of achievement.

A word of warning
It is not uncommon for people who have stopped smoking for some time to start again. Why is this? Some people just give in to temptation. These are usually people who have remained psychologically addicted to cigarettes. The other kind of lapsed ex-smoker is the one who thinks that an occasional cigarette will not hurt. **DO NOT MAKE THIS MISTAKE**. If you have been addicted before, it is very easy to become addicted again. The only way to eliminate this risk is to abstain from smoking **completely**. This means no occasional cigarettes, not even a puff.

Obesity and Cardio-vascular Disease
In addition to being a major risk factor for heart disease, obesity can also increase the likelihood of a wide variety of other conditions including diabetes, arthritis and certain forms of cancer. Being overweight or obese can have profound psychological effects too, and may cause considerable unhappiness.

Obesity is a common problem in the industrialized world, and despite growing health consciousness, it appears to be becoming more common in certain countries. For example, in England 39% of men and 32% of women were found to be overweight in 1980; in 1992 these figures had grown to 48% and 40% respectively. Now is the time to address the problem of obesity and its associated conditions.

What does being overweight or obese actually mean?
Overweight and obesity are both conditions in which there is an excess amount of body fat. The difference between them is merely one of degree, with obesity being the more serious condition.

How is obesity calculated?
Excess weight can be calculated in a number of ways. Probably the three most commonly used ways are the **body mass index**, the **body fat percentage**, and the **waist to hip ratio**. Each measurement looks at weight in a slightly different way.
Body mass index
The body mass index (BMI) is popular amongst members of the medical profession as a way of

The day you stop smoking should not be viewed with fear or trepidation; it is a reason to celebrate

> *Overweight and obesity are both conditions in which there is an excess amount of body fat. The difference is merely one of degree*

ascertaining the degree of an individual's weight problem. You can calculate your BMI by dividing your weight in kilograms by the square of your height in metres.

The higher your BMI, the heavier you are. The following is a guide to medically determined bands which relate BMI to the risk of ill-health.

The BMI looks at overall body weight in relation to height, and is therefore not a very good guide to body make-up. People who are heavily muscled may have a high BMI, but that does not mean they are fat. It is not being overweight that is the problem, it is being **over fat**. Ascertaining your body fat percentage (BFP) will help you to distinguish between what may be excess fat and a big build.

Body fat percentage

Body weight is made up of a number of constituents, including water, muscle, bone and fat. The parts of

the body other than fat make up what is termed the **lean body compartment**. This is relatively stable, and in healthy individuals makes up between 80% and 85% of body mass.

Body fat is sometimes described as **fat mass**, and although quite stable in some, can be prone to large fluctuations in others.

BFPs are normally calculated from skin-fold thickness measurements taken with callipers at various sites over the body. Ideal values for men and women are as follows:

♥ **Men:**   **10 – 21% of total body mass**
♥ **Women: 15 – 25% of total body mass**

If you are above these values, the higher your BFP, the greater your risk of all the chronic diseases associated with excess fat such as: heart disease, diabetes, hypertension, cancer and arthritis.

Waist to hip ratio

Fat is stored in different parts of the body to varying degrees. What is more, there tends to be quite a distinct difference between how men and women store fat. These differences seem to have important implications with regard to health.

Men tend to put weight on around their middles (above the waist). This is sometimes referred to as **abdominal** fat, and gives rise to a characteristically apple-shaped physique.

Before the menopause, women tend to put most weight on around the thighs and buttocks. This fat is sometimes referred to as **gluteal** fat, and produces a more pear-shaped figure.

Importantly, abdominal fat is strongly associated with ill-health, while gluteal fat appears not to be. In other words, the larger your waist is in comparison to your hips, the greater your risk of ill-health. We can therefore measure the **waist to hip** ratio to help us predict whether excess body fat is likely to be putting us at risk of illness.

Body mass index table

Each of the bands has a different implication for health:

BMI Men		BMI Women
less than 20	underweight	less than 19
20–25	healthy	19–24
26–30	overweight	25–29
31–40	obese	30–40
more than 41	very obese	more than 41

Underweight: *Being underweight is a relatively rare problem, and may be associated with an eating disorder such as anorexia nervosa. Those who are underweight may be at increased risk of ill health.*

Healthy: *If you fall into this category, then your weight is ideal. Your aim is to maintain this level of weight in the coming years.*

Overweight: *People who fall into this category may possibly have health problems as*

a result. There is a moderate risk of heart disease at this level of weight. Steps should be taken to reduce weight in the long term.

Obese: *Obesity is strongly associated with ill-health, and it is likely that anyone falling into this category will be at significant risk. Steps should be taken to reduce weight immediately.*

Very obese: *At this weight health is seriously at risk. Immediate action to lose weight must be taken.*

The ideal waist to hip ratios for men and women are:

♥ **Men: less than 0.95**
♥ **Women: less than 0.85**

Values greater than these are associated with factors such as reduced HDL ('good cholesterol'), hypertension, high total cholesterol, and a tendency to develop diabetes later in life.

Men and women really are different

Because men tend to store fat around their middles, and it is abdominal fat which is associated with ill-health, they are likely to suffer more than women as a result of their excess weight. However, it appears as though male fat has no real function, and the body is therefore quite happy to lose it. Because of this, men can often lose weight with relative ease.

Gluteal fat, although not associated with ill-health in the same way, does seem to have an important function physiologically. It appears that gluteal fat is designed to be used as an energy reserve during pregnancy and breast-feeding. It is probably because of this vital function that gluteal fat has been shown to be resistant to dieting. Women who have struggled to lose weight in the past may take comfort from the knowledge that the reason for this is simply a natural part of womanhood, and not a failing on their part.

The pitfalls of dieting

Many weight loss programmes are based around the principle that the fewer calories we eat, the more weight we lose. Although this principle works in most cases in the short term, there are important reasons why the effect cannot be sustained. What is more, long-term calorie restriction can put enormous strain on the body.

The calorie principle was first put forward in 1930 by two doctors, Newburgh and Johnston, at the University of Michigan in the US. Their original study was conducted over too short a period of time to draw any conclusion about the long-term effects of calorie restriction, but was nevertheless accepted as gospel by the medical establishment.

We now know that severe calorie restriction can have a number of harmful effects:

♥ Although the calorie principle works initially, the body soon detects that its food intake has been cut. In this situation, the body goes into starvation mode, and does everything it can to preserve the energy stores it has. This means the less you eat in the long term, the less your body will burn. This explains why many people's weight may plateau no matter how little they eat.

♥ Once you abandon a diet and start eating normal volumes of food, the body is suddenly unable to cope with the increased demand. Because of this effect, the weight that was lost quickly returns, often with a few pounds added on for good measure. Repeated cycles of weight loss followed by weight gain ('weight-cycling') have been shown to have an adverse effect on health, particularly with regard to heart disease.

♥ Losing weight on a strict diet does not mean you are losing fat. In order to make up for the food you are not eating, the body does not just break down fat to use as energy, it breaks down protein (muscle) as well. The last thing you need on a diet is to reduce your lean body mass. Conventional diets may lead to weight loss, but body fat percentages often change very little.

♥ Calorie-based diets place more emphasis on the quantity of food ratherthan the quality. Even an apparently healthy diet isunlikely to supply all the vitamins and minerals we need in the amounts necessary for peak health. When we begin to cut down on the amount of food that we eat, and at the same time eat foods which are low in nutrients (most diet

Weight loss programmes based around the principle that the fewer calories we eat, the more weight we lose work in the short term, but there are important reasons why the effect cannot be sustained

> *The body does not just break down fat to use as energy, it breaks down muscle as well – the last thing you need on a diet is to reduce your lean body mass*

foods are),we are in grave danger of suffering from the effects of vitamin and mineral depletion.

In other words, if you want to end up hungry, overweight and malnourished, go on a diet.

A sensible approach to weight loss

If you are planning to lose weight, then the best way to achieve this is through a sensible and healthy approach to your diet. We must think of our body as a furnace, with the fire representing our metabolism, and the fuel the food we eat. In order to keep the furnace burning we need to ensure that we use the right fuel, and put it on the fire on a regular basis.

In simple terms this means eating good quality food, and eating to a sensible pattern. Rubbish foods such as fast foods, sweets, cakes and confectionery are a bit like damp logs on the fire, they do not tend to burn very well. Fruits, vegetables and wholegrains like wholemeal bread burn much better.

Some people who are following diets think that skipping meals and going hungry must be the best way to lose weight. If we think for a moment about the fire inside us, then we can see just how mistaken this belief is. If we light a fire at breakfast time and do not fuel it at midday, what happens by the time we come back to the fire in the evening? The flame will be so low that the fuel we put on it in the evening will not burn easily at all. Skipped meals mean that our body is more likely to store subsequent meals as fat.

A basic guide to healthy eating

This ten-point guide to healthy eating covers the basics of good nutrition. More information about diet and nutrition can be found in chapter 7 (see p.67).

1 **Eat three meals a day.**

2 **Eat something healthy
if you get hungry between meals.**
Fruit is the ideal between-meal snack.

3 **Never skip meals.**
If time is short or you are eating on the move, eat a few pieces of fresh fruit.

4 **Drink healthily**.
The healthiest drinks are mineral water and freshly squeezed fruit and vegetable juices. Avoid caffeine (it stimulates your body to secrete insulin which can lower blood sugar). Soft drinks are full of sugar and/or artificial chemical additives, and are best avoided.

5 **Drink alcohol in moderation.**
A moderate amount of alcohol is compatible with a healthy diet. Moderate drinkers have lower mortality rates than teetotallers.

6 **Drink mainly between meals
and not at meal times.**
Drinking at mealtimes dilutes the secretions which digest food and therefore disturbs the digestion.

7 **Cut down on your intake of fat,
particularly saturated fat.**
When choosing protein rich foods, go for fish first, poultry second (remove the skin) and red meat last of all. When eating dairy products, go for the low-fat varieties wherever possible, e.g. low-fat cheese, skimmed or semi-skimmed milk and low-fat yoghurt.

8 **Choose unrefined carbohydrates.**
These include wholemeal or other 100% wholegrain bread, brown rice, potatoes in their jackets and wholewheat pasta. These foods contain far more in the way of fibre, vitamins and minerals than their more refined and processed versions.

9 **Avoid sugar.**
This not only means not adding sugar to food and drinks, but also means being wary of foods which have sugar added.

10 **Eat plenty of fresh fruits and vegetables.**
Vegetables are better either raw (e.g. salad),

steamed, or microwaved. These forms of preparation preserve more of the nutrients in the food than boiling, baking or frying.

Heart disease and food supplements

Oxygen is essential for life, and is involved in countless reactions in the body. However, our use of oxygen is not without risk. During such chemical reactions, **free radicals** can be formed. These are unstable atoms or small molecules which have can react with other compounds in an often dangerous, uncontrolled way. Free radicals can damage cells, with serious consequences. For example, the cells which line the coronary arteries try to heal themselves by plugging up the damage caused by free radicals with cholesterol and blood clots, thus increasing the risk of heart attack.

Because free radicals are dangerous, the body has developed ways of controlling them using substances to limit free radical production, or to limit the extent of their effect. Chemicals which control free radical formation are known as **antioxidants**, because they suppress oxidation which gives rise to free radicals.

There is some evidence to suggest that a diet rich in antioxidants may help protect against heart disease. Foods which contain high levels of these nutrients include wholegrains, fruits and vegetables. Dietary sources may be supplemented with zinc, copper, manganese, selenium, vitamins A, C and E, and beta-carotene in order to reduce free radical damage.

It is important to remember, however, that vitamin and mineral pills should be considered as supplements to and not substitutes for a basic healthy diet.

Diabetes and Cardio-vascular Disease

Diabetes mellitus or 'sugar diabetes' is a now recognized as the third leading cause of death in the US. Because diabetics often lead what appear to be active, normal lives, most people do not recognize diabetes to be the national health problem it is. Diabetes has seri-

Healthy meal suggestions

The following meal suggestions are examples of healthy options based around these principles:

Breakfast

Fresh fruit of any kind and in any amount.
Wholemeal toast with a thin spread of butter.
Mushrooms on toast with grilled tomatoes.

Lunch

Wholemeal avocado salad sandwich.
Jacket potatoes with coleslaw, salad and garlic mushrooms.
Chicken, tuna or prawn salad.
Lean beef or lamb with vegetables.
Vegetable soup with wholemeal bread.

Evening meal

Wholewheat pasta with tomato and mushroom sauce and salad.
Vegetable or chicken curry with brown rice.
Stir fried chicken with vegetables.
Steamed, poached, grilled or baked trout or salmon with vegetables.

Between-meal snack

Any fresh fruit or fruits.

ous and debilitating complications, and reduces overall life expectancy by about one third.

Most cases of diabetes are related to lifestyle, particularly obesity and lack of exercise. There is therefore a great deal that can be done to help protect ourselves from this condition.

Diabetes and sugar metabolism

To understand diabetes, it is necessary to know something about how sugar is handled in the body.

Carbohydrate is the main source of energy in the diet, and is made up of a range of substances from simple sugars at one end, to more complex structures composed of interlinked chains of sugar molecules at the other. Glucose is an example of a simple sugar, while starch is an example of a complex carbohydrate

Vitamin and mineral pills should be considered as supplements to and not substitutes for a basic healthy diet

found in foods like bread and potatoes.

When carbohydrate is eaten, simple sugars are absorbed into the bloodstream via the gut. Digestive enzymes are used to break down complex carbohydrates into single sugar molecules prior to absorption. As these molecules are absorbed, the blood sugar level starts to rise. The pancreas responds to this by secreting a hormone called insulin. Insulin facilitates the absorption of sugar into the body's cells, and this process is essential to the regulation of the blood sugar level.

Diabetes mellitus is a condition in which sugar metabolism is disordered and blood sugar levels tend to be higher than desired. The condition comes in two main forms. In the first one, the body produces insufficient insulin, whereas in the second, the body is resistant to its effects.

Type I diabetes

Type I diabetes usually comes on abruptly in childhood or adolescence. For this reason it is sometimes referred to as **juvenile-onset diabetes**. This type of diabetes makes up approximately 10% of all diabetics. The principal problem is that the body is unable to secrete insulin, and so the sufferer must inject insulin on a regular basis to control the blood sugar level. Insulin-dependant diabetes is another name for this condition because of this.

Scientists believe that Type I diabetes is a largely hereditary condition, and its development is unaffected by lifestyle factors such as diet.

Type II diabetes

Type II diabetes makes up about 90% of all cases of diabetes. It generally comes on slowly during middle or old age, and for this reason is sometimes referred to as **adult-onset diabetes**. The problem is not that insufficient insulin is produced, but that the body is resistant to its effects. Type II diabetics usually have normal or elevated levels of insulin in the blood.

Type II diabetics can normally control their condition with dietary modifications and/or oral medication. The term non-insulin dependant diabetes is used to describe this condition. However, insulin is sometimes used in these patients if these measures prove inadequate.

The effects of diabetes

A common complaint of diabetics is fatigue. This is because the body is not getting enough fuel. Even though blood sugar levels may be high, the cells are unable to absorb this sugar to convert it into energy. Other common symptoms include drowsiness, itching, skin infections (e.g. boils) and poor wound healing. Because the kidneys have to work hard to get rid of the excess sugar, more urine is passed than normal. Thirst is a common symptom as a result.

The long-term consequences of diabetes can be serious and life-threatening. These include:

- ♥ **Coronary heart disease.** A diabetic is two and a half times more likely to suffer from heart disease than a non-diabetic. Diabetes accelerates the process of atherosclerosis.
- ♥ **Stroke.** Stroke is more common in diabetics. (Heart disease and stroke make up three quarters of the causes of death in diabetics.)
- ♥ **Peripheral vascular disease.** Atherosclerosis in the arteries of the legs can lead to problems with circulation, ulcers and gangrene. Amputation is not uncommon.
- ♥ **Neurological problems.** Failed nerve function can lead to numbness, tingling sensations, impotence, diarrhoea and abnormal bladder function.
- ♥ **Blindness.** Diabetics are 25 times more prone to blindness than non-diabetics.
- ♥ **Kidney disease.** Diabetics are seventeen times more prone to kidney disease than non-diabetics.

Preventing and controlling diabetes

Type II diabetes is closely linked to obesity and inactivity. In fact, many experts believe that the majority of cases could be prevented through proper diet and exercise. We have already discussed the basics of healthy nutrition. However, it is worth focusing on one or two points which are particularly pertinent to the diabetic.

Diet and the diabetic

Because of recent findings in dietary research, some doctors are advocating diets for diabetics which are high in fibre and complex carbohydrates. This is to help ensure that sugar is absorbed slowly into the bloodstream, thereby reducing the demand for insulin.

The effect of fibre is to slow the rate at which food passes from the intestines into the bloodstream. A diet which is high in fibre will contain good amounts of wholegrains, fruit and vegetables. Such a diet will also contain essential vitamins and minerals.

Carbohydrates are absorbed into the bloodstream at different rates. In general, simple sugars are absorbed more quickly than the complex starchy carbohydrates. Sudden intakes of simple sugars can give rise to insulin surges which result in rapid reductions in blood sugar, often to levels below the ideal. Low blood sugar or **hypoglycaemia** is associated with symptoms such as fatigue, irritability, food cravings and headaches. Hypoglycaemia is common in women, particularly prior to a period.

Complex carbohydrates need digestion prior to absorption, and therefore tend to be released into the bloodstream more slowly. The rate at which sugar is released into the bloodstream can be quantified using a measure called the **glycaemic index**. Here, the rate of absorption of a food is compared with that of the same quantity of pure glucose which is assigned a glycaemic index of 100. Foods which are digested rapidly have a high glycaemic index (more than 50), while foods which are more slowly digested have a low glycaemic index (less than 50).

Interestingly, we find that whether a carbohydrate is complex or simple is not necessarily a good guide to its glycaemic index. Potatoes, which are traditionally thought to release sugar slowly into the blood, actually turn out to have a high glycaemic index, and therefore place relatively high demands on insulin. A table of the glycaemic indices of common foods appears above.

Chromium and blood sugar control

Chromium is an essential trace element, necessary for blood sugar control. Chromium is also thought to affect the way in which we deal with fats in the body, and can help lower blood fat concentrations.

Chromium deficiency, which is thought to be due at least in part to diets rich in refined carbohydrates (such as white bread and sugar), has been linked to a range of diseases including diabetes, heart disease and athero-

Glycaemic Index

Diabetics, and people wishing to minimize their risk of diabetes, should consume foods which have low glycaemic indices. Again, we can see that this will entail eating a diet which is rich in wholegrains, fruits and vegetables.

High Glycaemic Index			
glucose	100	chocolate bars	70
baked potatoes	95	sweetcorn	70
white bread	95	white rice	70
honey	90	boiled potatoes	70
cornflakes	85	non-wholewheat pasta	65
carrots, cooked	85	bananas	60
sugar	75	dried fruit	60
sugared breakfast cereal	70	jam	55

Low Glycaemic Index			
whole rice	50	whole cereals	35
wholemeal bread	50	fresh fruit	35
wholewheat pasta	45	lentils	30
oatmeal	40	chick peas	30
whole rye bread	40	green vegetables	less than 15
peas	40	tomatoes	less than 15
unsweetened fresh fruit juice	40	mushrooms	less than 15

A diabetic is two and a half times more likely to suffer from heart disease

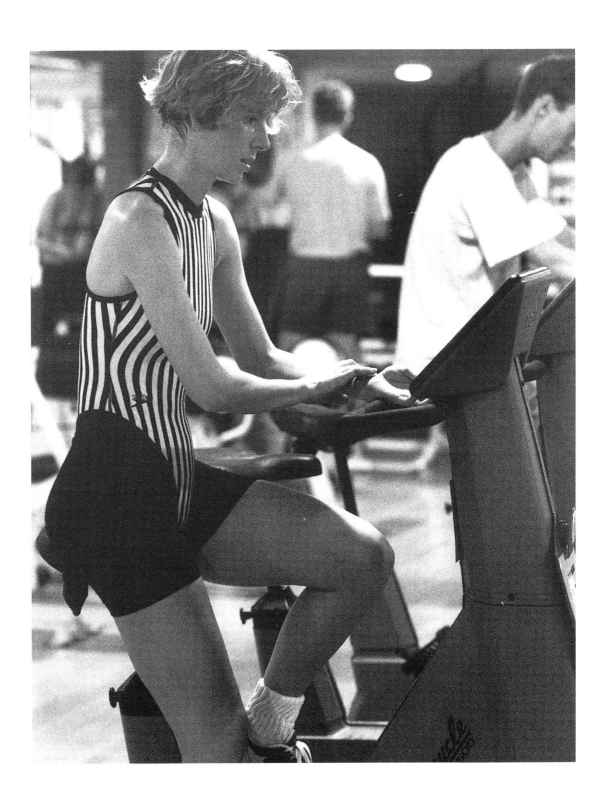

At the start of an exercise programme, you may need to experiment with taking your pulse quite often to make sure your heart rate is in the target range

sclerosis. These conditions are more prevalent in the Western world where there is an abundance of refined carbohydrates in the diet.

It seems that for chromium to be biologically active it must be combined with vitamin B3. This composite compound is known as glucose tolerance factor chromium or GTF-Chromium. GTF-Chromium is thought to bind to insulin and potentiate its effect. Chromium can therefore be a useful supplement in sufferers of non-insulin dependant diabetes.

Interestingly, GTF-Chromium seems to stabilize blood sugar levels, and can also help prevent hypoglycaemia. It can be a very useful supplement in women who suffer from premenstrual sugar and sweet cravings due to hypoglycaemia.

Additional supplements in diabetes

Other nutrients which may be of value in diabetes include vitamins C, B6 and B12 along with the minerals zinc, magnesium and potassium.

Exercise and Cardio-vascular Disease

It is now well established that regular exercise helps maintain and improve health and well-being. The benefits can be physical and mental, and range from reduced risk of heart disease and diabetes, to lower levels of stress, depression and anxiety.

However, very few of us do enough exercise to enjoy a health-related benefit. What is more, lack of exercise reduces our capacity for physical work, leads to less efficient heart and lungs, and causes reduced bone and muscle strength. Exercise, therefore, is an essential part of healthy living.

What are the benefits of regular exercise?

Regular exercise has been associated with a wide range of health-related benefits. These include:

- ♥ reduced incidence of heart disease
- ♥ improved bodyweight control and reduced risk of weight-related illness
- ♥ reduced risk of developing diabetes in later life
- ♥ enhanced muscle strength and joint flexibility
- ♥ increased capacity to cope with physical work
- ♥ reduced incidence of thinning bones (osteoporosis)
- ♥ reduced incidence of the symptoms of premenstrual syndrome
- ♥ reduced levels of stress, anxiety and depression
- ♥ enhanced mood and self-esteem.

In addition to the above, regular exercise has other important social advantages which can enhance the quality of life. Physically active individuals are more likely to live life to the full, well into old age.

How much exercise should I take?

When discussing how much exercise to take, we must consider three factors: the **intensity**, **duration** and **frequency** of exercise.

Intensity

Since the 1960s, the heart rate has been used as a measure of the intensity of exercise. It has been established that an exercise effort of between 60% and 80% maximum heart rate (MHR) is sufficient to gain fitness and health benefits. The MHR is the rate at which the heart rate peaks with maximum effort. It has been calculated that MHR can be estimated using the following formula:

♥ **Maximum heart rate equals 220 minus age**

The maximum heart rate for a 40-year-old is therefore 180. This equates to a target heart rate of between 108 and 144.

To find out whether you are exercising to the correct intensity, stop exercising for a moment to take your pulse. The pulse can be felt on the inside of your wrist close to the base of your thumb. Count the number of beats you feel in fifteen seconds, and multiply

> *It is now well established that regular exercise helps maintain and improve health and well-being*

> **Consistency is essential if you are going to enjoy lasting effects from the exercise you take...**

Calculating MHR the hard way on a stationary cycle at specific workloads and wearing a heart rate monitor.

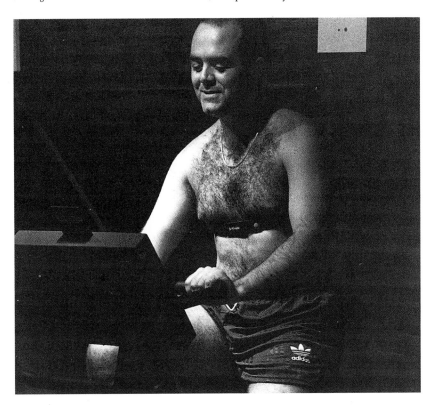

this figure by four to calculate your heart rate.

At the start of an exercise programme, you may need to experiment with taking your pulse quite often to make sure your heart rate is in the target range. In time, however, you should get a feel for the sort of level of activity needed to raise your pulse to the desired level.

Activities which are likely to raise your heart rate to the desired range include brisk walking, light jogging, vigorous swimming, cycling and trampolining.

New thoughts on exercise intensity

Researchers at the Ball State University in Indiana recently analysed a sample of over 2,000 people to test the accuracy of the conventional formula for calculating MHR.

The researchers looked at factors which may affect the MHR, and particularly what made it lower or higher than predicted. They discovered that older, lighter, non-smoking men and women tended to exceed the MHR predicted for age, while younger, heavier smokers tended to have an MHR well below the predicted value.

What this means is that the conventional method for calculating MHR may not be appropriate for everyone. There is a risk that some individuals, particularly the overweight and smokers, may be attaining target heart rates which are higher than desirable. For other individuals (e.g. the elderly, lightweight and non-smokers), the predicted values may be insufficient to give aerobic benefits from exercise.

An alternative approach for prescribing exercise intensity has been the Perceived Rate of Exertion (PRE) which was developed in Sweden in the 1970s. This requires that individuals exercise at a rate that is psychologically and internally assessed on a number of different levels.

The PRE scale is becoming increasingly popular in the gymnasium and sports training settings. The Indiana research suggests it may be of value, if not for everyone, then at least in those for whom the existing MHR formula may not be appropriate.

Duration

The question of how long it is necessary to exercise for benefits to be realized has been hotly debated over recent years. Most researchers tend to agree that 30 minutes worth of exercise is sufficient to contribute to aerobic fitness. Incidentally, it is after about 20 minutes of aerobic exercise that fat starts to be used as a fuel in appreciable amounts. Up to that point, energy is supplied almost exclusively in the form of glycogen, a starch-like substance which is stored in the liver and muscles.

A study conducted a few years ago at the Baker Institute in Melbourne, Australia, looked specifically at how much exercise was of most benefit in bringing down blood pressure. The results showed that exercise sufficient to raise the pulse to 120 beats per minute was most effective, as long as this was undertaken for 45 minutes, three times a week. Some experts advocate exercising for up to an hour at a time.

You are certainly going to benefit from aerobic exercise which lasts from 30 minutes to an hour, and it is likely that as long as you are not overstretching yourself, the longer you exercise for, the greater the benefit. However, it seems that after about 30 minutes, the amount of benefit to be had from any additional exercise you may take declines somewhat.

Frequency

One very important component of any exercise programme is frequency. Consistency is essential if are going to enjoy lasting effects from the exercise you take. It is generally accepted that exercise should be taken three to four times each week, or every other day. It is advisable to spread the exercise you take out over the course of the week. This will give your body time to recuperate in between the bouts of exercise, and therefore makes subsequent training sessions more manageable.

How do I start?

If you have not exercised for some time, then you must build your level of activity gradually. Probably the safest way to do this is to take brisk walks, lasting about half an hour, about three times a week. Gradually, you may wish to increase the intensity, duration and frequency of these walks. Eventually you can progress on to another, more strenuous form of exercise if you feel you are ready.

Whatever form of exercise you choose, it is important that you enjoy it. Exercise should not be some kind of penance or chore. If you do not enjoy what you are doing, you are unlikely to keep it up. Some people enjoy a sense of competition. Some people find exercise particularly enjoyable if they join a group or class. Team spirit can be a powerful motivator and may have other social advantages too.

Many people do not take enough exercise because they do not feel that they are the 'sporty' type. You don't have to be 'sporty' to reap the benefits of regular, healthy exercise. Whether you exercise alone or as part of a team or class, the effect is equally beneficial.

A word of caution

Exercise is a perfectly safe process for the great majority of individuals. However, some may have specific problems which need to be taken into consideration before commencing an exercise programme.

These problems include the following factors:

♥ If you are aged 40 or more, and particularly if you have any of the risk factors for heart disease, please consult your doctor before starting an exercise programme.

♥ If you have bone or joint problems such as a bad back or arthritis in your knees then the type of activity you take should be selected with great care. Discuss the matter with your doctor, osteopath, chiropractor or physiotherapist; he or she will be able to advise you about which types of activity are safe for you.

♥ Diabetics who do not require insulin are at no risk during exercise and should participate normally. Diabetics on insulin need to be more careful as their requirement for insulin may decrease. Insulin-dependant diabetics should consult their doctors prior to starting an exercise programme for this reason.

You don't have to be 'sporty' to reap the benefits of regular, healthy exercise

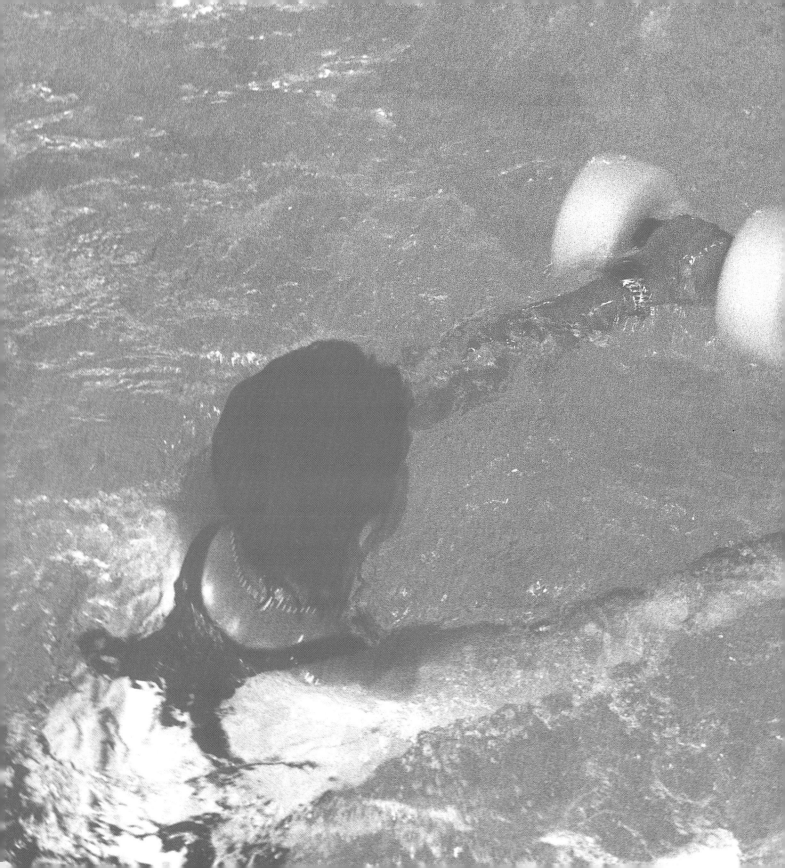

CHAPTER FOUR

CONQUERING CANCER

In the industrialized world one in three people will develop cancer at some point in their lives, and one in every four or five people will die from it.

There is almost certainly some genetic component in most forms of cancer, but in all probability, this is relatively small.

Lifestyle factors have an important influence on our risk of cancer. The World Cancer Research Fund estimates that about two thirds of all cancer deaths are related to smoking or diet. A commitment to healthy living can therefore go a long way towards protecting us from cancer and its effects.

What is cancer?

Cancer is not just one disease, but a collection of diseases, all of which have one common characteristic: uncontrolled cell growth and replication.

The body contains many different organs such as the brain, liver, kidneys, bowel, stomach and breast. Each of these organs is made up of millions of tiny components called **cells**. Different organs and tissues have different functions, so the cells in them are different too. For example, the cells which line the stomach are very different from those in the brain. In most tissues, cells are gradually 'turned over', with

> *About two thirds of all cancer deaths are related to smoking or diet*

old cells being replaced by new ones during the process of renewal. This is normally a controlled process, so that overall the tissues produce just enough new cells to replace the old, dead ones.

Cancer comes about when one cell begins to multiply uncontrollably. A group of abnormal cells is produced, which in time can form a tumour. The speed of growth of a tumour depends to some degree on the tissue in which it originated. The tissue which gives rise to a tumour can also determine the likelihood of that tumour spreading to other parts of the body.

Benign and malignant; what do these terms mean?

Tumours that are cancerous are often described as '**malignant**'. Malignant tumours have a tendency to spread, not only locally, but also to distant parts of the body. A cancer that has spread from an original site is known as a **metastasis** or **secondary**. The original cancer is sometimes also referred to as the **primary**.

Malignant tumours, if left without treatment, almost invariably prove fatal. Treatment is usually in the form of drug therapy (chemotherapy), radiotherapy, surgery, or a combination of these treatments. The aim of surgery is usually to stop the tumour from metastasizing or spreading, because once this has happened the tumour is, generally speaking, much more likely to be fatal.

Not all tumours are malignant. Many are not aggressive, and even though they can grow quite large, do not tend to invade local tissues or spread to other parts of the body. Such tumours are described as **benign**. Benign tumours are usually harmless and tend not to recur once they have been removed.

Is cancer curable?

Some cancers are more easily cured than others. What is almost universally true is that the earlier the cancer is diagnosed, the better the outlook and the better the prospects of a full recovery.

Cancer comes about when one cell begins to multiply uncontrollably

What causes cancer?

Because cancer is actually a collection of different diseases, there are a large number of potential causes. Risk factors for one type of cancer may not be the same as for another. For example, smoking is the main risk factor in lung cancer, but not in skin cancer.

However, scientists have now been able to isolate the following risk factors which may increase our risk of developing cancer:

- ♥ smoking
- ♥ dietary factors such as high fat and low fibre content
- ♥ excessive alcohol consumption
- ♥ obesity
- ♥ excessive exposure to the sun or ultra-violet light.

Each of these factors will be discussed with particular reference to cancer, and recommendations will be made about how we can minimize our risk.

Cigarette smoking and cancer

Smoking a packet of cigarettes a day increases our risk of lung cancer five fold. Lung cancer is responsible for **one quarter** of all deaths due to cancer. There is absolutely no doubt that smoking is the major, most easily avoidable cause of cancer in the West, particularly amongst men.

In addition to being the main cause of lung cancer, smoking also makes a number of other cancers more likely. These include cancer of the mouth, larynx (voice-box), oesophagus (gullet), stomach, bladder and cervix. Smoking is thought to have some of its effect through the production of free radicals, the rogue atoms or groups of atoms which were described in the section on cardio-vascular disease (see p.39).

Free radicals can disrupt the DNA inside a cell which controls its division, and this may lead to uncontrolled replication. There are over 50 chemicals which have been isolated in cigarette smoke which are known to be cancer-causing agents (carcinogens).

Stopping smoking is essential to minimize the risk of cancer. Advice about how to go about doing this is given in the section on smoking in relation to cardio-vascular disease (see p. 34).

Diet, alcohol and cancer

Experts who study the causes of cancer believe that a large number of cancer deaths could be prevented by making sensible changes to our diet. Many scientists believe a third of all cancer deaths are diet-related, and this has important implications for anyone wishing to reduce their risk.

The World Cancer Research Fund guidelines designed to lower cancer risk are:

1 Cut down on the amount of fat in the diet. This applies to both saturated and unsaturated fats. The proportion of energy in the diet derived from fat should be reduced from its current level of 42% down to 30%.

2 Eat more fruit, vegetables and wholegrain cereals.

3 Consume salt-cured, salt-pickled and smoked foods only in moderation.

4 Drink alcohol in moderation, if at all.

Each of these four aspects will now be discussed in more detail here.

Dietary fat and cancer

The amount of fat in the diet is linked with risk of cancer. This seems to apply particularly to cancers of the breast, colon, rectum, ovary and prostate.

The precise role of fat in cancer is not yet known, although some evidence exists to suggest that fats in the blood are important in promoting the growth of certain tumours.

Another possible mechanism to explain the link between fat and cancer relates to free radical formation. It appears that fats which are obtained from our diet are particularly susceptible to the action of free radicals. It is thought that fat molecules can be con-verted into highly toxic forms (called **trans-fats**) by free radicals, and these toxic fats may play an important role in the triggering of cancer cells. Supposedly, the greater the surplus of fat and oils over antioxidants in the body, the greater the risk.

Information about saturated and unsaturated fat, and advice on how to cut down your fat intake is given in the section on cholesterol in relation to cardio-vascular disease (see p. 27).

Fruit, vegetables, wholegrain cereals and cancer

Increasing the amount of fruit, vegetables and whole-grain cereals in our diets may help protect us from cancer. It is probably the abundance of fibre, vitamins and minerals in these foods which is responsible for their protective effect.

Fibre, the part of plant foods which humans cannot completely digest or absorb, reduces our risk of colonic cancer.

Some scientists believe that certain foods contain toxins or chemicals which may induce cancer in the lining of the colon. It is thought that by speeding the passage of food through the intestine, fibre reduces the time during which these chemicals can have their effect.

Vitamins and minerals play an important role in the fight against cancer too. Many of these nutrients have antioxidant properties, and help to control the free radicals which are implicated in cancer.

Some of the nutrients which are thought to be of particular value are:

♥ **Beta-carotene.** Beta-carotene is converted to vitamin A by the body, and is thought to protect against several cancers, particularly cancer of the lung. Beta-carotene is abundant in fruits and veg-etables that are deep yellow or orange in colour, such as carrots, sweet potatoes, peaches, apricots, oranges and bananas.

The amount of fat in the diet is linked with risk of cancer

> *Maintaining a healthy body weight seems to be important in reducing our risk of cancer*

♥ **Vitamin A.** In laboratory studies, vitamin A has been shown to protect against several cancers. However, it can be toxic, should be avoided in pregnancy, and is best taken under medical supervision.

♥ **Vitamin C.** May protect against some types of cancer, such as cancer of the oesophagus and stomach. Good sources of vitamin C: broccoli, cauliflower, green peppers, strawberries and citrus fruits.

♥ **Vitamin E.** Early evidence suggests that vitamin E may help protect against cancers of the oesophagus and stomach. Vitamin E is found in wholegrain cereals and unsaturated vegetable oils.

♥ **Selenium.** Studies have shown a strong inverse relationship between the mineral selenium and cancers of the breast and colon. It may be that healthy amounts of selenium in the diet can protect against these, and other cancers too. Good sources of selenium include grain, fish and most wholefoods.

Salt-cured, salt-pickled, smoked foods and cancer

Eating large amounts of salt-cured, salt-pickled and smoked foods has been linked to cancer of the oesophagus. The smoke from curing seems to create carcinogens in the food, while salt-cured and salt-pickled foods contain chemicals which can be converted into carcinogens in the food or in the stomach.

Grilling or barbecuing food over an open flame can also create carcinogens on the surface of foods, particularly if the food is charred and fatty.

Should the above foods make up a substantial part of your diet, you may benefit from cutting down on their consumption.

Alcohol and cancer

The consumption of alcohol appears to increase the risk of developing certain forms of cancer. In moderate amounts, alcohol seems to be linked to an increased risk of cancers of the breast, rectum and pancreas. In excessive amounts, especially when combined with cigarette smoking, alcohol may also increase the likelihood of cancer of the mouth, oesophagus and larynx. Heavy drinkers who have cirrhosis of the liver are more prone to liver cancer.

To a degree, the link between cancer and alcohol is confused by the fact that individuals who drink quite a lot of alcohol are more likely to smoke and to have poor diets. How much is due to the alcohol itself and how much is due to these other factors is in doubt.

The information given here about alcohol and cancer must be balanced by emerging evidence about the correlation between alcohol and overall mortality. This was touched on in the section concerning alcohol, heart disease and mortality (see pp. 30-31).

Obesity and cancer

Women who are overweight or obese appear to be at increased risk of cancers of the breast and uterus (womb). Studies also suggest that obese men may have increased likelihood of cancers of the prostate and colon. The reason for these findings is still not entirely clear, though they may well have something to do with dietary factors such as levels of fat and fibre consumption. *Maintaining a healthy body weight seems to be important in reducing our risk of cancer.* Advice about losing weight through healthy eating is given in the section on overweight and obesity in relation to cardio-vascular disease (see p. 35).

The sun and cancer

The relationship between sunlight and skin cancer has been publicized a great deal in recent years. In general, the advice from cancer specialists and dermatologists has been to limit exposure to the sun, to use sunscreens and shading devices, and to avoid burning.

In some quarters, the precise link between sun and skin cancer is hotly debated.

Skin cancer

Skin cancers make up about 10% of all cancers. There are actually several different forms of skin cancer, some more serious than others. The three main types are: **basal cell carcinoma**, **squamous carcinoma** and **malignant melanoma**.

The basal cell and squamous varieties together make up 98% of all skin cancers. Their relationship with sunlight is clear; they usually occur on the exposed surfaces of the body such as the face, the scalp, and the back of the hands. They are common in the elderly, particularly those who have lived for some time in the tropics. It is likely that long-term steady exposure to sunlight is what triggers these cancers, but chances of survival are very good. Ninety-five per cent of individuals are alive five years after diagnosis.

Malignant melanoma, which is very rare, is more serious. Only 50% of patients are alive five years after diagnosis. This compares reasonably favourably, however, with cancers in general, which have an overall five-year survival rate of about 36%.

However, the case for the link between sunlight and malignant melanoma is not as clear cut as the one linking it to the other skin cancers.

Sunlight and cancer in general

Several studies have claimed that exposure to sunlight actually protects against cancer. When the rate of cancer deaths for different parts of the world are plotted against latitude, the lowest death rates occur in regions closest to the equator. People who live in higher latitudes, e.g. Scandinavians, seem to have about two and half times the risk of those at lowest risk. There is a case for sunlight being protective against cancer in general.

Some scientists believe that this phenomenon may be explained by the fact that certain cancers, e.g. cancers of the breast and colon, have a correlation with high socio-economic status and socio-economic status is related to latitude. The debate continues.

Sunlight, skin type and melanoma

There is a particularly high incidence of melanoma in Queensland, Northern Australia, one of the hottest, sunniest parts of the world. This fact has probably promoted the belief that melanoma is caused by exposure to sunlight and sunburn. However, a large study was performed in 1984 in Western Australia examining 507 melanoma cases, comparing them to 507 individuals without melanoma who were matched for age, sex and place of residence. The study found that *people who regularly spent ten hours per week* or more in the sun *were less likely* to develop malignant melanoma, and *the longer the time spent each week in the sun, the lower the risk*.

In 1985 research from Canada suggested that the real risk of melanoma comes not from sunburn, but from having *a type of skin that burns easily*.

Research into the incidence of skin cancer in the US concluded that in temperatures over 42 degrees centigrade, increases in exposure to sunlight caused an increase in **all types** of skin cancer, but below that temperature, the rate decreased with increasing exposure to the sun.

It seems that in hot, tropical climates there is a risk of sunlight causing skin cancer, particularly in those who have fair skin. However, in more temperate climates, sunlight may actually protect us from cancers.

> *The study found that people who regularly spent ten hours per week or more in the sun were less likely to develop malignant melanoma*

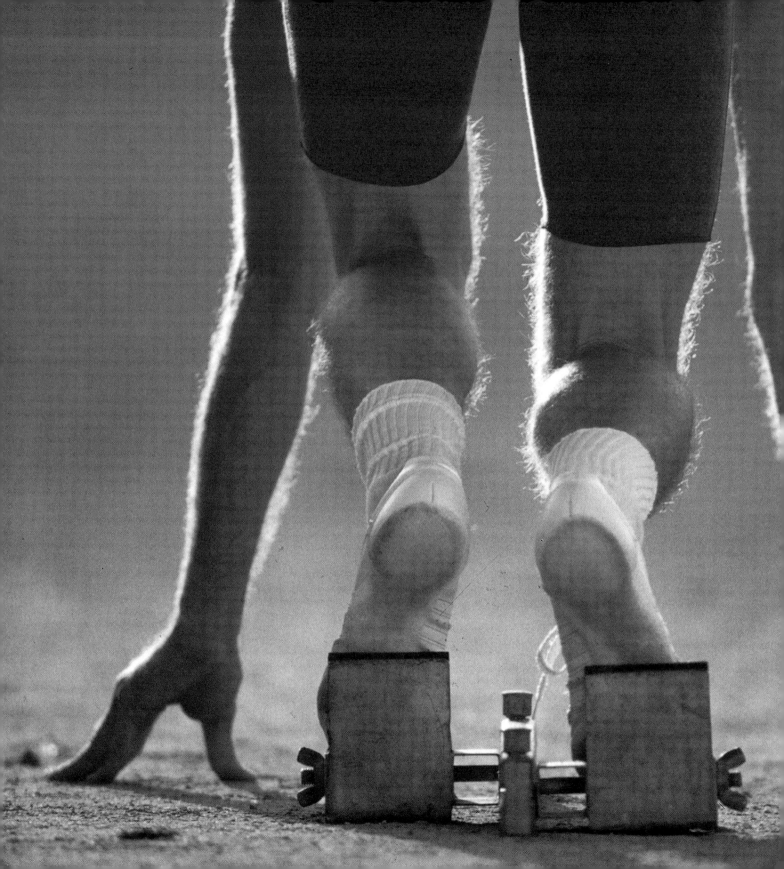

C H A P T E R   F I V E

THE JOY OF STRESS

Most people worry about stress.

They look upon its darker side as though stress were synonymous with distress...

Take, for example, two people driving quickly in a car – one can be exhilarated by the speed and danger, the other terrified by it. Their physiological responses would have been almost identical. Both hearts would have raced and pounded, their blood pressures undoubtedly were significantly raised, their muscles tensed, their breathing quickened and so on.

But one enjoyed the experience and was stimulated, the other was deflated and depressed.

The variance arises from the psyche of each individual. Figure 4 overleaf illustrates the physical reactions which actually take place.

Stress itself occurs in four different ways:

1 **Actual physical discomfort** – too hot, too cold, windy, etc., through to applied torture or wounding.

2 **Anticipation** – parachuting, making a speech, being interviewed, before a sporting contest or examination.

3 **Unanticipated** – a sudden accident or near-miss, a fright.

> *The stress of anticipation is often greater than the event itself*

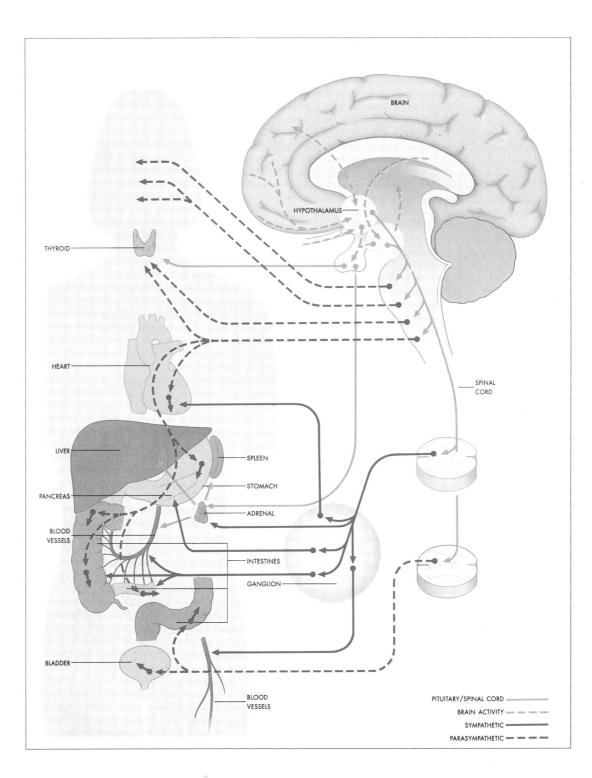

Our imagination can heighten anticipatory stress

Figure 4

4 **Frustration** – one or a series of unpleasant occurrences beyond the control of the stressed individual.

Sometimes one kind of stress follows another – for example, the physical injuries sustained in a mugging or accident. In some, the stress of anticipation is often greater than the event itself. Research found parachutists were more anxious before jumping than actually during it. Scientists at the US Air Force School of Medicine measured pulse rate and hormone secretion in subjects about to receive a pin prick and found often the mere expectation of pain was enough to generate all the stress symptoms in the body even if the needle never touched the skin.

The same anticipatory stress can be used as a motivation in sport. Once the competition starts, most contestants can usually relax and concentrate on their game or event.

Examinations, too, cause anticipatory stress and can motivate and stimulate some people whilst terrifying and depressing others.

Basically, stress affects us in three ways: *emotionally, behaviourally and/or physiologically*. It can be negative or positive. It all depends upon our approach, our ability to self-analyse and to accept inevitability.

Some businessmen boast they promote stress in others rather than suffering it themselves. These are the deliberate stress-makers. Most athletes fall under this category. They become addicted to competition and seek other outlets even after they retire from their prime sport.

The recent and most famous example of all is that of Michael Jordan who, upon retiring from an outstanding basketball career during which most judges acclaimed him as the greatest player in history, almost immediately turned out to play baseball. People find it difficult to understand how he can be bothered playing in Triple A minor league baseball in front of a few hundred fans for a very low salary when he was earning millions as a basketball player competing with the Chicago Bulls in front of sell-out crowds of 20,000.

He is also renowned for high-stakes golf matches. A substantial number of top sportsmen gamble – the stress it promotes is in their blood.

Of course, the lure of the bet is not restricted to them. Millions get their 'kicks' from anticipating correctly the throw of the dice, the turn of the card or the speed of the thoroughbred.

Extreme stress-seekers are the bungy-jumpers, the mountain climbers, around-the-world sailors, the arctic explorers and so on. There are literally hundreds, perhaps thousands of ways to add anticipatory and physical stress to one's life.

The greatest basketball player of them all, Michael Jordan, retired from the sport which paid him millions, but continued to feed his addiction to stress by taking up minor league baseball.

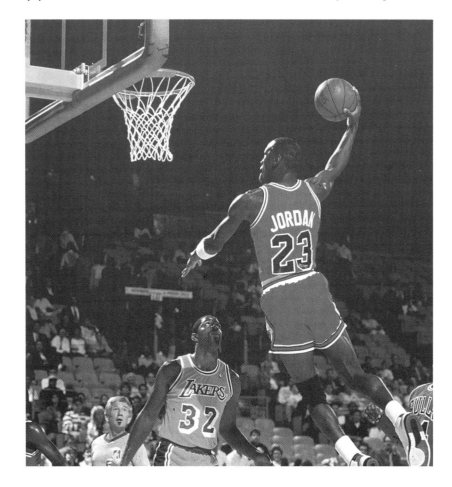

'Not for me!' you say. 'I can live very well without any stress whatsoever, thank you very much!' you claim. But can you?

In fact, some stress is necessary to well-being. Scientists relate that when experimenting with animals, they were able to eliminate all forms of stress. The results were that the animals became completely erratic in their behaviour; they appeared to go mad or they simply withered away and soon died.

Lifetime workers look forward to retirement away from their day-to-day stress-loaded routine only to physically sicken from boredom when the time comes.

The latest medical evidence is :

♥ a lack of stress can be harmful
♥ stress itself should not have any harmful aftermaths on the body or the heart
♥ without stress most physical and cultural occurrences would be mundane.

On the other hand, it is acknowledged that severe stress can :

♥ cause serious ailments
♥ make people accident-prone
♥ have disastrous consequences.

It really all depends upon how you are able to cope with it.

Coping with stress

Hans Selye worked for 50 years at the Institute of Experimental Medicine and Surgery at the University of Montreal. From his introduction to the effects of stress as a nineteen-year-old medical student in Prague, he devoted his life to its study and research.

Born in Vienna, he headed the University's research into stress and became the foremost expert in the field. It was he who named the sequence of the body's reaction in the process of physiological stress – the *general adaptation syndrome*. His theory was that everybody naturally possessed an unreplenishable store of 'adaptation energy' to control stress, but this remains unproven. The more stress with which you had to cope, the lower your reserves became.

With his experiments on animals, particularly with rats, Selye worked out a detailed sequence of behaviour he claimed was the routine aftermath of stress.

Firstly, there is the *alarm – the fight or flight stage*, then the *resistance or coping stage* and finally the stage of *exhilaration or breakdown*, the extreme result of which is death. According to Selye, death occurred when the animal exhausted its 'adaptation energy' reserves. It was unable to alter its behaviour to accommodate the continuing severe stress.

When the animal was dissected it invariably had:

♥ enlarged adrenal glands
♥ shrunken lymphatic nodes and thymus
♥ a lowered immune system
♥ a stomach with bleeding ulcers.

In man, where the mind is so powerful an agent in the body's mechanism, often this sets up a psychological barrier to save the physical presence at the cost of mental stability.

Man's ability to think and reason both relieves and heightens stress reactions. For example, stress of physical discomfort can be overcome by shedding or adding clothing, by sheltering in the wind, by bathing if humid, or stopping if tired.

On the other hand, our imagination can heighten anticipatory stress. Invariably, the reality is not as frightening as expected. And if we think clearly we can always take some action to relieve our frustration about another's lack of understanding.
No psychological expertise is claimed here, but we put forward some suggestions for your consideration should you be feeling over-stressed.

1 Regard stress as a stimulant rather than a depressant and either:

> **Man's ability to think and reason both relieves and heightens stress reactions**

a Acknowledge and accept situations you cannot control, setting out solutions in writing for various sets of circumstances which may befall, from the very worst to the best.

b Make your choice between fight and flight and move on to the next stage, if necessary, as soon as possible.

c Resistance is the automatic consequence of the former. If you decide to fight, then you should make certain you do so fully prepared and reconciled to all possibilities including failure (without becoming too negative).

d Communicate with others, or a particular trusted confidant, your fears and doubts, frustrations and anger, even seeking their advice as to the merits of your various options. But if you ask for advice, listen carefully to it without debate. You may not choose to follow it; but once asked your friend deserves a full hearing and you may hear some angle you had not previously considered.

e Hopefully very few people will be faced with frightening situations not of their making, when resistance is apparently futile and 'fight or flight' is not an option. Abject subjugation may do something to relieve a ghastly situation. Despite the loud and frequent protestations of the macho set, surrendering to fight or fly when circumstances are more favourable, is not a bad alternative to consider and accept when, for the moment, these are impossible.

2 Break the pattern causing the stress
either by exercising, meditating, travelling or simply doing something different. Physical exercise of some sort, or a yoga class combining exercise with meditation and breath control can work wonders. But holidaying, changing routines, even clothes, residence or eating habits can all relieve stress.

3 Analysing the type of stress
and your options and the stage of 'adaptation', can help concentrate your thoughts on the best solutions in given circumstances. Remember:

a There are four different ways stress occurs: *physical*, *anticipation*, *unexpectedly* and by *frustration* (not in control), but although physiologically our bodies react in the same way, our mental ability to cope with stress varies.

b There are three types of *effect: emotional*, *behavioural* and *physiological*, and we should be analysing how we are being affected, to what degree and how deeply, as by knowing and recognizing the cause and effect of any deviation in our emotions, behaviour or physical well-being, we should be able to plan and effect our recovery.

c There are three stages of stress on the body and mind: *fight or flight*, then *resistance* and finally *exhaustion* or *exhilaration*. We should establish at what stage we are, and how to avoid the situation deteriorating further.

The message is there is nothing to fear but fear itself, seek to analyse, communicate and to relieve and, if at all possible, enjoy – after all, to repeat, without stress life is inconsequently dull.

Of course, the fitter you are physically, the more likely you will be able to cope with stress situations – fight, flight or resist become a challenge of choice, an election rather than a reaction.

Even the physiological effects, such as racing of the heart and increased blood pressure, become a pleasant rather than an unpleasant experience for the fit person – after all, exercise itself extends the body's ability to resist these reactions and to keep them within acceptable limits. You become familiar with the feeling.

Then again, if you literally have to fight, run or struggle you are physically far more able to do so – but we hope we can all avoid such occurrences with the exception of fair and acceptable sporting events and competitions.

Lastly, we would like to remind you of that old Boy Scout motto 'Be Prepared'. It is sensible advice.

> *Of course, the fitter you are physically, the more likely you will be able to cope with stress situations – an election rather than a reaction*

Yoga is not a religion but a philosophy, although it developed in the monasteries and ashrams of the East

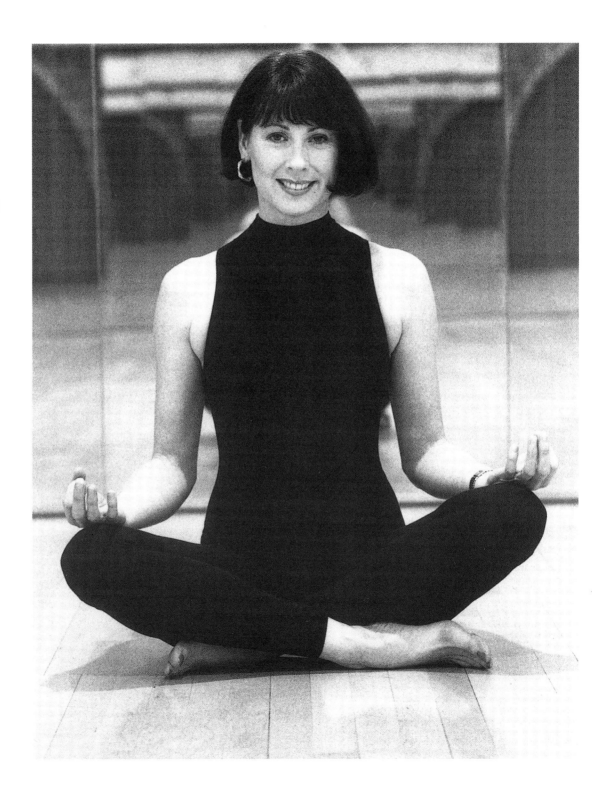

The beauty of yoga

There are many misconceptions about yoga. Firstly, it is not a religion, rather a philosophy, although it developed in the monasteries and ashrams of the East. The word *yoga* means 'union' and, basically, treats both the body and the spirit (or mind) in the belief that, until the physical being is healthy, supple and free from illness and disease, the mind is not free to pursue its goal of union with the divine or *atman* which it is believed lies within each human being.

Many forms of yoga have developed. Our concern is with Hatha yoga, the yoga of physical health which combines *asanas* (firm postures), *pranayama* (the control of breath), *krigas* (movements repeated rhythmically) and *mudras* (neuro-muscular stimulation to pressure glandular secretions) combined with relaxation techniques to produce total health of mind and body.

There are certain rules your yoga master will insist on. In summary, usually these are:

1 Clean the body by showering *before* your session.
2 Practise yoga early in the morning or at least four hours after eating so your stomach is empty – *this is important.*
3 Yoga *asanas* are best done on the floor, using a firm, clean pad and sheet in an airy, quiet site, free from all distractions.
4 Do not wear belts or scarves or other restrictive clothing – your hair should be short or tied back.
5 You should be prepared to practise every day. Like all physical activities which are worthwhile, progress is slow and steady – *this is no short-term activity if you really wish to benefit.* Neither will you find instant results or gratification but if you are prepared to devote sufficient time and attention, consistently, then the benefits are immense.

There is a special diet – actually, fairly normal principles, closely linked to the Hay Plan which we reiterate in chapter 7 (see p. 97).

Your teacher will probably begin by instructing you in your breathing patterns. Yoga devotees are convinced that breathing properly enhances the whole spectrum of physical activity. Breathing is divided into four phases – inhaling, suspension, exhaling and a further suspension.

There is no doubt that mastery of breathing rhythms can dictate and control an infinite range of physical and emotional actions and reactions.

Only after learning about breathing will you be shown the various yoga stances which improve flexibility, posture and health so much.

Hand in hand with your breathing control and those stances come the relaxation techniques.

Finally comes the training of the mind and the methods of lapsing into meditation.

We strongly recommend to anyone who feels they have the time to at least undertake a three-month introductory course of Hatha yoga. Should you not wish to continue on a fully committed basis, the knowledge and techniques you will have acquired will assist you greatly in your physical and emotional well-being.

> *Yoga devotees are convinced that breathing properly enhances the whole spectrum of physical activity*

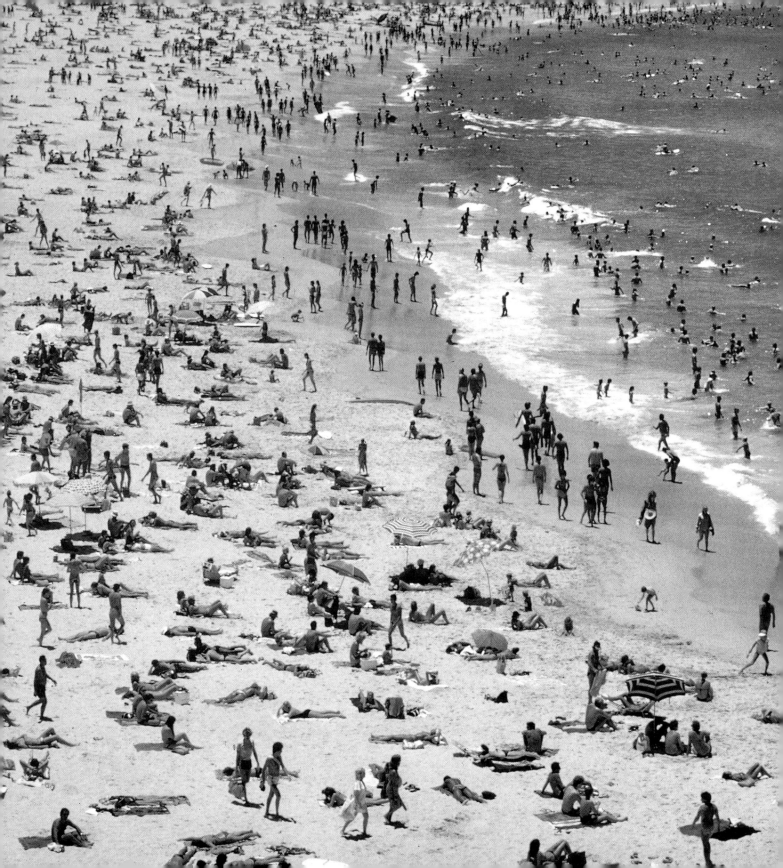

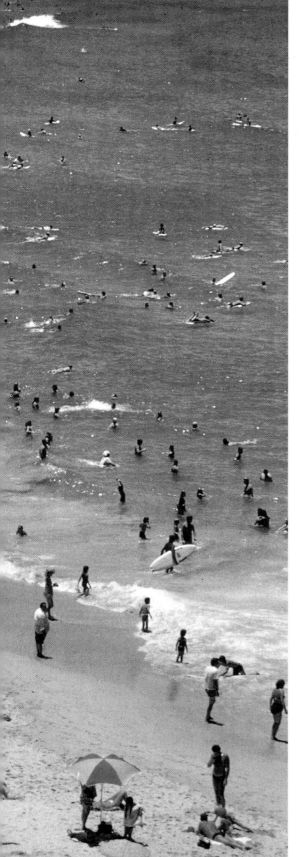

CHAPTER SIX

THE SUN: SAINT OR SINNER?

I have always been a sun-lover.

My earliest recollections are the beaches around the bay in Melbourne, running and trotting around bare-headed or bare-chested after my brother and father.

This latest fad in Australia of avoiding the sun at all costs, of covering up outdoors to escape the evil aftermath of exposure to ultra-violet rays has completely bemused me.

Australian kids used to be thought so fit and healthy with a glorious all-year glow to their cheeks and a liveliness in their eyes.

Now, for the main, they are as pale and dull-eyed as their British cousins.

The trend reminds me of the publicity given at the outset of the jogging craze by orthopaedic surgeons. *'Our practices have increased three- or four-fold from injuries to the knees and joints being incurred by all those fools out there pounding the streets'*, they said.

What they had not taken into account was that there were ten to twenty times the number running

Now, for the main, they are as pale and dull-eyed as their British cousins

> *Skin should be gradually conditioned to ultra-violet rays of the sun over an extended period, and avoiding the midday hours*

the streets than previously, so a three- to four-fold increase was disproportional anyway. What was even more important, their colleagues, the cardiologists, were simultaneously commenting on the general improvement in health which was becoming apparent in their field because of the increased numbers of people jogging regularly.

Right now the dermatologists have the floor 'down under' with their alarming reports on the increasing number of skin cancers they are encountering. But are they necessarily putting together the correct cause and effect? This chapter takes a closer look at ultra-violet radiation with its benefits and consequences.

I have always understood the skin should be gradually conditioned to ultra-violet rays of the sun over an extended period, and avoiding the midday hours.

If, as happens nowadays, many more hours are spent indoors than out, then when exposure does take place it will be more likely to burn an unprepared skin and this, rather than the exposure itself, may increase the risk of skin cancers because it is a sun burn and not a sun tan which causes the problems.

I think that *Slip on a shirt! Slop on the sunscreen! Slap on a hat!*, the Australian-made television commercial slogan, now universally accepted by virtually everyone out there as gospel truth (no Australian will go into the sun nowadays without slip, slop and slapping), is fine, provided it is applied sensibly. But surely it should be balanced by some publicity on the benefits that ultra-violet can have on people's general health; this would encourage the sensible enjoyment of one of the world's most wonderful resources.

At Cannons, situated in the heart of grey, overcast London, we like to feel our ultra-violet solariums provide an essential service to those office workers trapped in an environment almost devoid of sunlight (even in summer).

The following advice we give to all our people. We are indebted to the research undertaken by Dr Damien Downing and published by Arrow Books in

1988 under the title of *Day Light Robbery*. I recommend this publication to anyone who has doubts about the benefits of sunlight.

One truism he stresses and which I recommend to my fellow Australians is:

'The evidence is that regular doses of sunlight help in preventing most cancers. It is sun-burning not sun-tanning that may cause skin cancer. To live all year indoors and then to fry on holiday is comparable to taking all of one's yearly intake of alcohol in a fortnight.' This is surely self-evident.

It is absolutely astonishing in these days of much greater awareness of the importance of our environment and natural products that the life-source of nature itself – the ultra-violet rays emitted from the sun – receives such bad press.

Without daylight, and the ultra-violet rays sustaining it during this period, life on earth would die.

As I have discovered, it is possible to go for months during winter in the United Kingdom without seeing a glimpse of the sun. We travel to work before sunrise, spend all day indoors, then travel home after sunset. Weekends can be spent mainly indoors and the few minutes we may spend outside rarely coincide with the very few hours of the week in which the sun actually appears through the constant cloud cover.

Even walking from the car, train or bus to work is usually via shaded streets.

In Western society, degenerative diseases are much more common than elsewhere in the world – including depression and other psychiatric problems. Is this simply our poor diet?

Dr Downing produces overwhelming evidence that living in temperate climates, with their low levels of sunlight, and then spending most of our time indoors is as important or more important a factor in the proliferation of these diseases, as poor nutrition and exercise levels.

But what about cancer?

Sunlight is a killer is the clear message from the

medical profession, especially in Australia but latterly repeated throughout the world.

Actually, you are less likely to die from cancer if constantly exposed to the sun or high doses of ultra-violet rays.

Here are two graphs showing, Table A, the cancer deaths per 100,000 population and, Table B, cancer deaths in the USA in terms of exposure to sunlight.

The benefits of vitamin D, the main natural source of which is sunlight on the skin, are numerous.

For example:

♥ It is the best and most effective way to lower blood pressure.
♥ It increases the uptake of calcium thus strengthening bones and preventing the onslaught of arthritis.
♥ It appears to give a significant protection against bowel cancer.
♥ It protects against and relieves the pain of rheumatism.
♥ It assists in the digestive functions of the intestine and in the efficient and healthy operation of the kidney.
♥ And most interestingly, it assists in the efficient circulation of oxygen through the blood vessels enhancing aerobic capacity by as much as 20%.

But, you may say, surely skin cancer and skin deterioration, as related in almost all the popular women's magazines and periodicals, inevitably follow exposure to the sun.

The answer is an emphatic **NO!** Sun-tanning, in fact, protects the skin and has many more beneficial effects. Sun-burning, particularly on celtic complexions, is the danger and can easily be avoided.

To quote Dr Downing: 'In the UK one quarter of all deaths are due to cancer. There are about 200,000 new cases of cancer every year, and of these about 10% are skin cancers. This breaks down to 98% squamous and basal cell cancers, and 2% melanomas.

But the chances of surviving skin cancer are excellent: 95% of patients are alive five years after diagnosis. This compares with a 36% survival for cancers in general. So, if you have to get cancer, then skin cancer is definitely the choice.

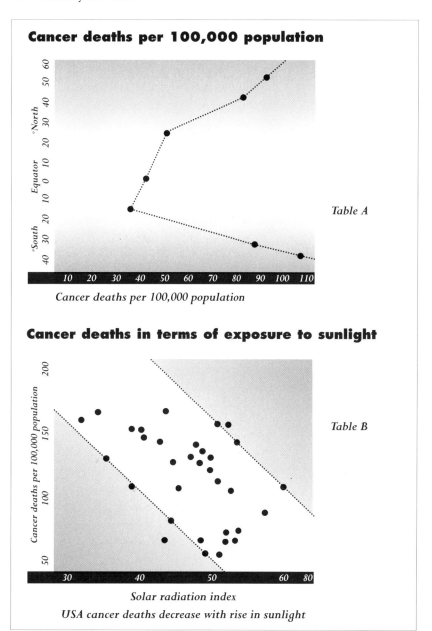

Cancer deaths per 100,000 population

Cancer deaths per 100,000 population

Table A

Cancer deaths in terms of exposure to sunlight

Cancer deaths per 100,000 population

Solar radiation index

Table B

USA cancer deaths decrease with rise in sunlight

The one big exception is melanoma, of course. Although it is very rare – about 0.2% of all cancers – it is the only skin cancer that normally metastasizes (spreads to distant parts of the body), and the death rate is much higher. The five-year survival rate is 50%, much poorer than the other skin cancers.

It still doesn't rank in the top ten killers, but if it were avoidable by simply staying out of the sun, this would plainly be a sensible thing for us all to do.

He then goes on to quote a number of studies which seem to contradict the generally held belief that the greater the exposure, the greater the risk.

One study, for example, which was carried out in Western Australia during 1984, found that '... If anything, exposure to sunlight protected against melanoma. People who regularly spent ten hours a week or more in the sun had a lower chance of developing the disease, and the longer time they spend in the sun each week the lower the risk.'

On the other hand, protection against cancer, and skin degeneration in general, relies on monitoring a healthy DNA and other molecules. UVA exposure enhances healthy DNA strands and repairs any damaged cells.

Dr Downing concludes that the medical evidence is clear that we, as with all plants and animals, are designed to feed on sunlight, and we suffer if starved of it. Changes in our lifestyle are drawing us indoors; to rectify this by brief binges of sunlight may well have harmful effects which offset these benefits, particularly if you have the wrong skin type.

The aim should be to nourish ourselves with sunlight regularly, every week of the year.

As long ago as 200 BC the benefits of the sun were known and appreciated. Greek athletes trained naked out of doors exposing all their muscles to its beneficial effect. Not so long ago sick children, old people and hospital patients were whisked out on to sunny balconies to aid their recovery; the arrival of the multistorey hospital put an end to that.

I firmly believe in the benefits of sunlight on the development of stamina and health and it is a fact that every male distance running record set in the last decade has been achieved by athletes who were born and lived all their lives in tropical climates – men from Kenya, Ethiopia, Mexico, Algeria and Morocco. Surely this is no coincidence.

I'll go further and predict that just as surely as no pale-skinned athlete has set any sprint records for 50 years except at altitude, no competitor born and bred outside the tropics will set a distance running record for the coming five, maybe ten, decades.

The effects of ultra-violet radiation on physical fitness

Regular exposure to UVA has a remarkable effect on the average office worker, and there are the considerable benefits it provides to the power, endurance and recovery time for athletes in training.

In 1945 two researchers, Dr R.M. Allen and Dr T.K. Cereton, did a study, entitled Effects of Ultra-violet Radiation on Physical Fitness, *at the University of Illinois. A group of generally unfit students were put on a physical education course. One half of the group were treated with ultra-violet light on a regular basis (group A) and the other half did the same exercise but did not get any ultra-violet radiation (group B). The results were quite emphatic.*

	Group A	Group B
Pulse rate after exercise	*Improved by 10 beats per minute*	*Improved by 3 beats per minute*
Recovery time after exercise	*Improved by 30%*	*Improved by 10%*
Muscular fitness	*Improved by 22%*	*Improved by 15%*
Cardio-vascular fitness	*Improved by 19%*	*Improved by 1.5%*

All subjects reported an increase in their enthusiasm for classwork, but one side effect of interest not included in the original scope of the experiment was that those in group A suffered only half the number of colds of those in group B, the control group.

The mechanics of the benefits when the skin is exposed to ultra-violet radiation or sunlight lies in the effect it has on the blood circulating just below the skin's surface. In reality, it is a further version of the famous Knott technique in which the blood is removed, irradiated with ultra-violet and then re-injected. The capacity of the blood to carry oxygen goes up within an hour and lasts for several weeks, in some cases by as much as 50%.

There is also a marked improvement in the level of glycogen stored in the muscle tissue for some extra hours after exposure to UV (although for 60 minutes immediately after treatment the glycogen levels drop).

So the lesson is, whilst sun-bathing or having a sun-lamp session immediately before any physical effort, especially any aerobic based event, is negative, if the session takes place during the afternoon or evening before the event, it could be very beneficial.

In parallel with the increase in glycogen stores goes a decrease in blood sugar or, more correctly, a normalization of abnormal blood sugar.

With abnormal blood sugar levels (such as experienced immediately after a cup of strong tea or coffee) we often become twitchy and tense, even agitated and aggressive, whereas too low a level results in feelings of depression, emotional crying fits, drowsiness, and even to migraines and irritability.

Regular doses of UV normalizes these levels to such an extent that it has been proven to help control the blood sugar levels of diabetics.

The other most positive effect regular doses of ultra-violet radiation has on the body is the pineal gland, the famous third eye, which regulates our whole hormonal balance.

It is now clear that it is this gland which produces melatonin in response to darkness. Melatonin promotes drowsiness and sleep.

The pineal gland also regulates the output of the pituitary gland which, in turn, produces hormones that control all the other endocrine glands, and thus every cell in the body. Most importantly, a healthy pineal gland assists in the whole rhythm of sleeping and working so important in all of us.

Research by Cornileus Ralph in New York in 1983 found that the administration of pineal extract to rats increased their lifespans by up to 25%.

Even weight control is greatly assisted by a pro-perly-functioning pineal gland because of its effect on basal metabolic rate.

We would therefore submit that all the evidence points to sunlight, or ultra-violet rays, rather than being something to be avoided, are essential to looking and feeling better. Fitness in general and cardio-vascular fitness in particular are greatly enhanced. We are able to build healthier muscles with greater endurance, to use up more calories more efficiently and to burn off fat deposits. Nothing improves the appearance and texture of our skin more than a gentle tan. We look more attractive, too, with a glowing, healthy skin and a slim, vigorous figure.

However, in between the benefits, one rule must be remembered when commencing or continuing with any ultra-violet radiation, be it from natural exposure to the sun, or from indoor solariums. It is '**do not get burned**'. Adopt a sensible approach, taking into consideration your skin type, and the degree of expo-sure your skin has had during the past month.

Sunburn may not be the root of all evil as some doctors and alarmists would have us believe, but it definitely does age the skin and release free oxidizing radicals into the body.

If we are exposed to sunburn repeatedly over many years, then it CAN lead to skin cancer. So avoid it. Just do not burn and all the remarkable benefits of the sun are yours – for free.

No competitor born and bred outside the tropics will set a distance running record for the coming five, maybe ten, decades

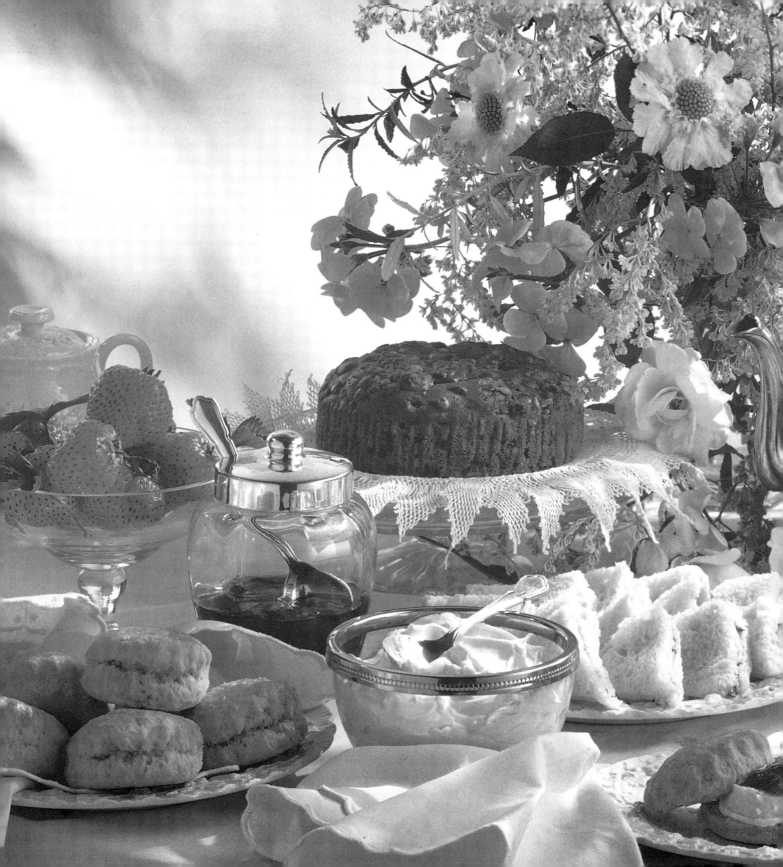

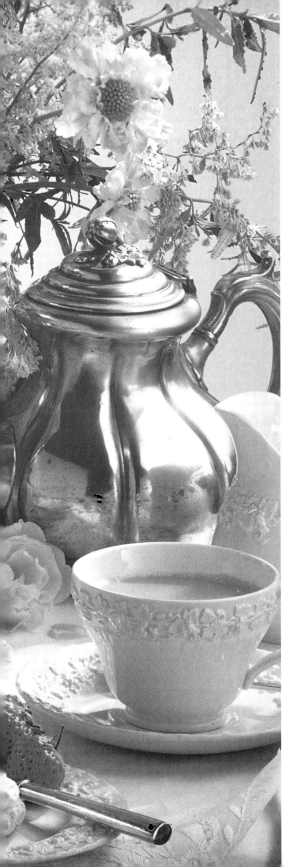

C H A P T E R   S E V E N

WEIGHT LOSS

JUST FOLLOW THE RULES

There are a few simple rules

to follow if you wish to lose inches and weight.

1 You should not starve yourself – never less than 1,000 k/calories daily for women or 1,400 k/calories for men.

2 These calories need to be balanced in what we call a 20:30 formula –

20% protein
but you can have a little more (up to 30%)
30% fat
never more but maybe less (down to 15%)
50% carbohydrate
or at most 55%.

It is easier to just remember 20:30 – and this is the basis upon which, since 1984, Cannons have been

Cannons have been 99% successful with our six- to eight-week weight loss courses

> *The key to any programme is discipline and knowing what nutrients are contained in which foods*

99% successful with our six- to eight-week courses averaging losses of four inches around the waist, and 12 lbs to 15 lbs off total net weight. Some of the participants have lost up to 25 lbs during just the 42 days of the shorter course (and have been able to keep it off afterwards).

3 Remember, when buying food, to apply the 4–9–4 multiples. That is:
- ♥ 4 calories for every gram of protein,
- ♥ 9 calories for every gram of fat, and
- ♥ 4 calories for every gram of carbohydrate.

4 Exercise is an important element. It does not have to be too gruesome. In fact, it should be fun. But if you want to trim and stay that way, exercise is inevitable.

Getting the fundamentals right

The success of any diet relies on balance – actually two simple balances.

Firstly, ensuring your food and drink intake is balanced as to its protein, fat and carbohydrate content. And, secondly, the kilo calories you consume should be less than your body expends.

Imbalance your diet too much, one way or the other, and unpleasant secondary repercussions occur. So, an all-protein diet can deprive you of energy for simple daily tasks and be as ineffective as a sub-1,000 k/calorie one. Too little fat, or a no-fat diet, encourages the body to convert its carbohydrate into fat which it stores.

There is no need to go to these extremes.

We will now show you how to go about organizing your own BEP – balanced eating programme – or, if you prefer, we can provide you with some options you can follow which have proven themselves at Cannons.

The key to any programme is discipline and knowing what nutrients are contained in which foods. If you can take the trouble to teach yourself what these are in the foods you and your family like and generally eat, then you have acquired the skills to control your weight from now on and into the future.

All you have to do is be smart and balance your diet by occasionally checking your total calories for the day. You do this best by writing down everything you eat, including the servings. Then calculate the calories and work out the percentages of the various nutrients from the grams consumed. This way you get to see for yourself what you are doing correctly … or wrongly.

Opposite you will see a sample format for a 'calorie tracer'. At Cannons, all those who participate in our 20:30 weight loss programme are shown how to use these calorie tracer cards and, for every day of the course, they are asked to calculate their daily k/calorie intake, and the percentages of protein, fat and carbohydrate.

All we ask you to do is to be aware. At least they try working it out for just a few weeks, after which you start to know the right amounts and types of food automatically. You balance your menus.

As someone once said – there is no such thing as a free lunch. If you want to indulge yourself consistently, then do not expect to be able to exercise it all off; accept you will be fat.

But if you can cut down to the odd rare binge you will enjoy it more when you do lash out and you will be able to control your health, shape and sanity much more effectively.

The time to start is now. Do not procrastinate; as we keep on saying, **Tomorrow Starts Today**. What you do today sets the mould. Delay and you will keep on finding more reasons to put off the start date.

Getting started

We do not offer miracles, so be warned – results are not going to be immediate. It is like building a 5,000 piece jigsaw puzzle. Whilst you are fitting the first few pieces in place the end result looks a million

Day				Date				
Food	Weight ounces	Weight grams	Descriptive measure approximate	K/cal	protein g	fat g	carbo- hydrate g	total

> *If we exercise more, or eat less, we lose weight. If the reverse happens, we gain weight. That's nature's law and nothing can alter this, whatever may be claimed*

weeks away, but you can only reach it by finding more pieces to go on the ones you have started. It is impossible to reach a result if you have to start fresh each week or so. But, keep at it for a while and you start to see the picture emerging, progress becomes discernible and encouraging, the right pieces are easier to find, the game becomes more enjoyable. Then suddenly presto! The whole picture is completed and you find it difficult to remember the trouble you were having getting started.

So it is with getting slim, whatever your reasons.

In fact, so consistently but subtly do the pounds come off and the measurements decrease that participants find it hard to remember what they were like when they started the course. For four to five years, we always took 'before and after' photographs to show exactly the remarkable transformation which came to those completing our courses.

It is important to realize that it is physically impossible to spot-reduce. If you have a large what's-it, the cause can either be hereditary, and nothing can change that, or because too much adipose (fat) has accumulated in that particular area (and even this can be hereditary – for example, if your parents tend to put on weight around the waist or hips as they get older, in all probability you will too unless you take steps to keep your overall weight level down).

We are what we are – our genes form our basic shape and dieting-cum-exercise programmes can only trim, tighten and slightly mould our outlines.

Fundamentally weight control is based upon a simple formula of balancing energy expenditure with food intake. The scientific method of measuring both these activities is the calorie, usually expressed in terms of kilo-calories (k/calories).

So, simply put, to maintain weight our daily exercise routine (expenditure) expressed in k/calories should exactly equal the calories we take into our body through what we drink and eat each day. If we exercise more, or eat less, we lose weight. If the reverse happens, we gain weight. *That's nature's law and nothing can alter this, whatever may be claimed.*

Our daily energy is helped along though by the fact we burn calories just by existing. We burn them while we sleep, sit, talk, sun-bake or generally leap around – usually more than 1,000 k/calories each 24 hours are consumed in this way.

This is called the basal activity or resting metabolic rate (RMR). To this we can add the actual exercise we do. Unfortunately, as we get older our RMR slows down so 50- and 60-year-olds, for example, can exist on less food than they have become used to eating during their 30s and 40s. The very old, in fact, often do lose their appetite and eat less but usually during our 30s, 40s and 50s, most of us continue to maintain the same eating habits, and thus put on weight because our RMR is dropping even if we are just as active as ever (which we rarely are).

So, it is a double whammy – our metabolic rate slows, we eat as much (or more) and exercise less (or less vigorously).

Therefore the odds are three to one our waistline will begin to thicken. Fat is insidious and accumulates slowly. At any one time a lean, fit athlete (with about 10% body fat) will have 60,000 calories of stored fat in his/her body. Imagine the enormous reserves of fat being stored by the normal 50-year-old male with a body fat percentage of about three times this – the norm is 27%.

So, by the time we reach 50 the chances are that these calories of stored fat have ballooned, without anything like the same need, to three times as much (around 200,000 calories) or to 30% of total body weight from the 10% or so we had, or should have had, when we were 20. There is no reason, except laziness, why this should not be brought back under control, to say 13% (17% for women), for the good of our health, our prospects of longevity, and simply to improve our day-to-day performance.

Nature has so arranged it that we have other requirements from food than fat for energy.

Carbohydrates also provide quick energy, whilst protein builds and repairs essential muscle tissue. To repeat, the ideal balance for food intake is about 20% protein, 30% fat and 50% carbohydrates – protein can form up to 25%, or carbohydrates 55%, but fat should not exceed 30% – in fact, it could drop to 25% or even 15%. These figures should become a part of your sub-conscious so that you can instantly recall them any time you are looking at a BEP.

To calculate your daily intake simply remember that protein and carbohydrate have four calories to each gram, whilst fat has nine calories to the gram.

So, to follow the rules of correct nutrition remember three simple sets of numbers :

1 20–30–50 **for the food elements**
2 4–9–4 **for conversion**
3 1,000–1,400 **for the minimum daily intake of calories.**

Why 1,000 calories? Because below this figure the body switches from consuming spare fat for its energy requirements to burning up its lean muscle tissue (so-called brown fat cells). So, instead of benefiting by losing more fat, you are actually losing muscle tissue whilst retaining your spare fat cells. As it is the percentage of your body made up of muscle tissue which sets the basal metabolic rate, by dieting and burning this off with a daily intake under the 1,000 calorie level, you are lowering your basal activity metabolic rate. Consequently, you will add fat more quickly once you begin eating normally again.

The result is that you stop dieting and you put on weight (fat) even more quickly than you did before – the dreaded yo-yo effect which afflicts many dieters.

In the pages which follow we will explain these principles in more detail but remember when you are reading them that *the fundamentals are simple if you remember the rules.*

There are no age restrictions – no reason at all why you should not be checking your daily intake, and bal-ancing this against your energy expenditure regularly, whatever your age. It is a lot more important to your future and general well-being than your bank balance, yet the people who wisely check their bank statements constantly, plan their expenses so they do not exceed their income, never bother to take the same trouble with their own health … and what use is all the money in the world if you cannot enjoy it?

To paraphrase an old Chinese philosopher: Intake 2,500 calories, expenditure 2,499, result: trouble. Intake 2,500 calories, expenditure 2,501, result: happiness. (That is provided, of course, the intake is properly balanced nutritionally.)

One of the aims of the diet recommendations in the Cannons 20:30 weight loss programme which follows is to familiarize you with a pattern of healthy eating that you can continue after the programme has ended; however, the main aim is for you to lose weight and inches. This means adhering rigidly to the calorie restrictions given.

The Cannons 20:30 Weight Loss Programme

Controlling weight is not just about calories. It is essential to achieve the correct balance of the following nutrients :

1 Protein
2 Fat
3 Carbohydrate – fibre
4 Vitamins – minerals.

What are these nutrients and why do we need them? Here is a simple analysis of the role of each…

Protein

Proteins are made up of amino acids of which eight are essential and must be provided in the diet. They are needed for the growth, maintenance and repair of body tissue. Protein is also needed for the synthesis of

> *It is a lot more important to your future and general well-being than your bank balance*

> *Saturated fat in particular, when eaten in large quantities, is a major risk factor for the development of heart disease*

hormones and enzymes. There is always some loss of protein from the body every day and so the diet must provide enough to replace this and to maintain the tissues.

There are two types of protein foods:

a animal protein
   – e.g. meat, offal, poultry, cheese, etc.
b vegetable protein
   – e.g. beans (baked, kidney, etc.), peas, lentils, nuts, bread.

Animal protein is of a higher quality because it contains more of the essential amino acids, and so it is important that on a calorie restricted diet, when levels of protein are also restricted, that a good proportion of the protein is high quality. But, in so doing, it is also important to make sure that you choose the lower-fat types of animal protein, such as lean meat, low-fat cheese, etc.

Fat

The basic units are triglycerides (glycerol base and three fatty acids). The major chemical difference between saturated and poly-unsaturated fats is that the former have single bonds and the latter double bonds within the carbon structure.

Fat is a source of energy but also provides fat soluble vitamins and the essential fatty acids which play important roles in membrane structure and hormone synthesis.

In dietetic terms, fats are divided into two groups :

a visible fats – e.g. butter, margarine, oils, etc.
b non-visible fats – e.g. meat fat, cheese, cream, pastries, etc.

Any diet must reduce fat in order to reduce the calories. Also, fat, saturated fat in particular, when eaten in large quantities, is a major risk factor for the development of heart disease. In the UK a recent survey found fat formed the largest portion in the average

daily diet of the population, more than both carbohydrate and protein. This is the underlying factor in the ill-health of the nation. Cholesterol is also a type of fat but it does not effect actual blood cholesterol as profoundly as saturated fat. Cholesterol intake automatically decreases when fat is reduced in the diet.

Carbohydrate

Carbohydrate should provide the majority of energy in the diet but in the UK people tend to consume less carbohydrate and more fat than they should. Carbohydrate can be divided into two groups:

a complex carbohydrates
b simple carbohydrates.

Complex carbohydrates

These are made up of long chains of single molecules joined together to form polysaccharides. They usually exist in an unrefined state and contain certain valuable vitamins, minerals and dietary fibre – e.g. wholemeal flour and bread, wholegrain cereals such as shredded wheat, brown rice, etc.

Simple carbohydrates

These are single or double molecule sugars and are found in large quantities in highly refined foods. They are often known as 'empty calories' as they provide energy without other nutrients – e.g. sugar, jam, sugary drinks and squashes, sweets, biscuits, jelly, etc.

Complex carbohydrates should be the carbohydrates of choice in a BEP because they are digested more slowly, thus providing a constant stream of energy which helps ward off hunger pangs. They also give the feeling of satiety and provide essential fibre.

Vitamins and minerals

A dietary regime should also be designed to provide all the vitamins and minerals required for health so that supplements will not be necessary.

Our Balanced Eating Plans

The BEP we recommend you follow is closely based on the recent recommendations for healthy eating from NACNE (see below).

We in the UK eat too much fat, sugar, salt and also too little fibre.

The state of the British diet prompted the publication of two reports:

♥ **COMA**

Committee on Medical Aspects of Food Policy

♥ **NACNE**

National Advisory Committee on Nutrition Education Report on recommended guidelines for healthy eating.

A combination of their recommendations is as follows:

1 Increase the proportion of carbo-hydrate in the diet to 50% – primarily complex carbohydrates.

Reason: To replace energy that will be lost when we decrease our fat and sugar intake. Also to provide more dietary fibre.

2 Increase our fibre intake to 30g/day.

Reason: A low fibre diet is linked with diseases such as colon cancer and diverticular disease. A higher fibre intake may protect against these diseases. Dietary fibre also helps keep blood cholesterol levels lower and gives a feeling of satiety which is useful when trying to lose weight.

3 Decrease the percentage of energy from fat to 30%, with saturated fat providing only 10% of the total.

Reason: Death rates from coronary heart disease in the UK are amongst the highest in the world and are linked to a high fat diet. Evidence has shown saturated fat raises the level of cholesterol in the blood and increases the risk of coronary heart disease.

4 Decrease sugar consumption to 20 kg/year.

Reason: Sugar provides 'empty calories' and is a major factor in the causation of obesity. It also contributes to the development of dental caries.

5 Decrease our salt intake to 9g/day.

Reason: A high salt intake is linked to the development of hypertension and this is another risk factor for coronary heart disease.

6 Decrease alcohol intake to 4% of total energy.

Reason: Alcohol, if taken in excess, provides an over abundance of energy and can lead to conditions such as liver cirrhosis.

The ultimate diet is thought to consist of 30% fat, 15% protein and 55% carbohydrate. However, our BEP contains a larger proportion of protein – 20%.

This is to ensure there is sufficient protein on these calorie restricted BEPs necessary for the additional exercise we also recommend to you as a part of the programme. When the programme is over you can increase your carbohydrate proportion and decrease your protein percentage if you wish since, in actuality, your body will probably be receiving the same amount in grams of protein as your total calorie intake will be returning to normal.

By decreasing the total amount of fat in your diet, you will also be decreasing the amount of saturated fat consumed. Saturated fats are found in animal fats, in meat (beef, lamb, pork, suet, lard and dripping) and in dairy products (milk, cheese, and butter).

Poly-unsaturated fats are found in sunflower, corn and soya oils, poly-unsaturated margarines, nuts and oily fish. So when you do eat fats, try to choose ones high in poly-unsaturated fat.

The sugar and salt content of your diets should also be reduced.

Here are some suggestions for doing this.

The best ways in which to decrease your intake of sugar:

♥ Drink tea or coffee without sugar. Use a sweetener instead if necessary.

The ultimate diet is thought to consist of 30% fat, 15% protein and 55% carbohydrate

> *Dietary fibre helps keep blood cholesterol levels lower*

♥ Choose low-calorie diet drinks and unsweetened fruit juices, e.g. Diet Pepsi, etc.

♥ Buy tinned fruit in natural juice rather than syrup.

♥ Avoid breakfast cereals with lots of added sugar.

♥ Avoid cakes and biscuits.

♥ Have fresh fruit rather than sweets or chocolates.

The best ways in which to decrease your intake of salt:

♥ Use a little salt in cooking but add no more at the table.

♥ Flavour foods with herbs or spices, rather than salt.

♥ Cut down on salted meats and fish, e.g. bacon, gammon, salt beef.

♥ Use fewer tinned and packet soups.

Alcohol

Alcohol should be avoided when on a calorie restricted diet. However, when you are not restricting calories, the level to drink is:

Men: 4–5 standard drinks 2–3 times per week

Women: 2–3 standard drinks 2–3 times per week

One standard drink is the equivalent of ½ pint ordinary beer, one measure of spirit, a small sherry or a glass of wine.

How do we make these changes?

Not all these changes may be necessary to convert your current diet into one nutritionally balanced but here is a plan to correct the various elements should you find it necessary to do so.

1 How to increase your intake of complex carbohydrates:

♥ Eat more cereals, bread, fruit and vegetables.

2 How to increase your intake of fibre:

♥ Choose wholemeal bread instead of white (brown bread is not the same as wholemeal).

♥ Use wholemeal flour in baking.

♥ Eat wholegrain breakfast cereals. There are many on the market, e.g. Weetabix, Shredded Wheat, Sultana Bran, etc.

♥ Try using more peas, beans and lentils in casseroles, soups and stews. In some meals some of the meat can be replaced with beans. Baked beans are a good source of fibre.

♥ Eat potatoes baked or boiled in their skin.

♥ Try wholegrain rice and pasta rather than the white varieties.

♥ Eat more fruit and vegetables which have some fibre, although not large amounts, but they do provide valuable vitamins and minerals.

3 How to decrease your intake of fat:

♥ Use a low-fat margarine or spread.

♥ Use skimmed or semi-skimmed milk instead of ordinary milk.

♥ Use low-fat yoghurt instead of cream.

♥ Use low-fat cheese, e.g. Shape, cottage cheese, edam, camembert.

♥ Use fish or chicken instead of red meat.

♥ When you buy meat choose the leanest cuts and trim off any fat. Remove skin from poultry.

♥ Avoid crisps, chocolate, cakes and biscuits.

♥ Grill instead of frying.

♥ Remove excess fat from mince using a spoon during cooking.

4 How to decrease your alcohol intake:

Avoid it completely, or follow these tips:

♥ Extra-dry drinks are lower in sugar and calories than sweet ones.

♥ Use low-calorie mixers.

♥ Add mineral or soda water to wine or fruit juice (lasts longer and reduces overall calories).

♥ Alcohol-free lagers and beers are low in calories.

Balanced Eating Programmes

So, why don't you, now, with the advice you have just read, write down:

a the normal daily diet of you and your family (maybe two or three typical days, one of which should be a weekend during which eating habits often change dramatically) – be sure that you accurately estimate the servings of each item and that you include snacks and nibbles you eat during the day. Then:

b using the advice offered to date, write down the same diet modified to meet the recommendations we have made, adding and restricting according to your particular tastes. Include servings that you think will satisfy you.

You now have two lists of two to three days' food and drink intake, including all snacks and extras; the first, what you *were* eating, and the second, adjusting this to the sort of diet you feel would be okay for you and your family. Draw down the pages six vertical lines to form five columns. Use our Ready Reckoner (see pp. 89–94) or a special reference book (we recommend and follow the *Collins Gem Calorie Counter*) to calculate in column 1 the k/calories of each serving. Then, in columns 2, 3 and 4, add the grams of protein, fat, and carbohydrate of each food item. At the foot of the page, or after the day's menu, add up each column and convert them into k/cals by applying the formula of 4 k/cals for each gram of protein or carbohydrate and 9 for each gram of fat. Then, add 2, 3 and 4 across to a total in column 5. Lastly, using that total in column 5 as a 100%, calculate all percentages of the other columns.

Do this for your normal and amended diets and compare them. How do the totals look? Can you cut some down if they are still too high (around 2,500)? If you really need to reduce these, they should come down to around 1,200 k/cals per day for women and to 1,500 for men. Do the relationships between the nutrients work out approximately correctly and, especially, is the fat content now under 30%? Perhaps you can reduce these by adjusting some of the servings. Compare these, perhaps, with some of the sample BEPs on the following pages in which we have already calculated the grams and various percentages. We strongly recommend you to design your own eating programmes – say four or five for variety – write them down and stick to them for six weeks. Otherwise, use ours.

You will note we also have listed some 'exchanges' on the pages following the sample BEPs which you can use to substitute one or two of the original items if they are unavailable, unsuitable, or you tire of them.

If you eat out, employ our Ready Reckoner, and write down your meals that day, repeating your calculations and seeing what penance you need to pay in order to balance out your intake again.

It really is that simple and not at all hard and fast (provided you maintain the balance) as you do have so many choices. First, do as we ask or follow our recommendations. Exercise as well (see chapter 8, p. 103) and your weight will consistently evaporate.

There are some sophistications regarding food balances, allergies and combining various types of food which we discuss on the pages following sample BEPs and our Ready Reckoner.

Snacks

Two of any of the following items can be eaten at any time during the day in addition to the day menus.

♥ Celery – unlimited
♥ Carrot sticks – unlimited
♥ Medium dates – 2 only
♥ Apple – medium
♥ Orange – medium
♥ Dried apricots – 2 only
♥ Dry popcorn – microwaved
♥ Raw cauliflower – 4oz
♥ Pumpkin seeds – 15g.

We strongly recommend you to design your own eating programmes – say four or five for variety, write them down and stick to them for six weeks

BALANCED EATING PLAN NO.1: DAY'S MENU

	K/CAL	PROTEIN (g)	FAT (g)	CBH (g)
Breakfast				
Either: Tropical breakfast shake	200	10.0	1.9	46.8
1 slice toast (wholemeal)	65	2.6	0.8	12.5
½ teaspoon margarine	20		4.0	0.1
Cup of tea or coffee				
A	**285**	**12.6**	**6.7**	**59.4**
Or: Banana	87	1.1	0.3	22.5
4oz low-fat yoghurt	85	10.1	8.2	13.1
2 slices toast (wholemeal) – dry	130	5.2	1.6	25.0
Cup of tea or coffee				
B	**302**	**16.4**	**10.1**	**60.6**
Lunch				
Either: Roast beef or tuna				
(water packed)				
or turkey sandwich with:				
2 slices of reduced calorie bread	80	2.6	0.8	13.2
½ teaspoon margarine	20		4.0	0.1
Sliced tomato	23	1.1	0.3	4.5
1 lettuce leaf	4	0.3		0.6
1oz low-calorie cheese (1½ slices)	21	2.7	0.8	0.6
2oz lean sliced roast beef; or				
½ can (7oz size) water-based tuna;	168	20.1	9.2	0.0
or 2oz roasted turkey				
No salad dressing				
Cup of coffee or tea				
Freshly-squeezed orange juice (4oz)	57	0.8	0.2	14.6
A	**373**	**27.6**	**15.3**	**33.6**
Or: Tuna salad:				
7oz size can of water-based tuna	114	25.2	0.8	
Bean sprouts, celery, pepper,				
onion, tomato, lettuce	35	2.0	0.5	4.5
Hard-boiled egg	72	5.6	5.2	0.3

No.1: Day's menu

	K/CAL	PROTEIN (g)	FAT (g)	CBH (g)
Lunch cont.				
Low-fat dressing	60	0.1	6.6	3.0
2 crackers	85	1.4	3.3	12.5
Cup of tea or coffee				
Freshly-squeezed orange juice (4oz)	57	0.8	0.2	14.6
B	**423**	**35.1**	**16.6**	**34.9**
Evening meal: Dinner				
Either: Mandarin chicken	228	30.2	9.7	
Baked potato (small)	72	1.8	0.1	17.1
Either salad: chopped lettuce	8	0.6		1.2
tomato	23	1.1	0.3	4.5
low-fat dressing	60	0.1	6.6	3.0
Or steamed vegetables:				
broccoli, carrots, tomato and peas	80	2.2	1.2	8.0
1 slice calorie-reduced bread	40	1.7	0.5	8.5
½ teaspoon margarine	20	1.2	1.5	7.3
Bowl of low-calorie soup	45	1.2	1.5	7.3
Cup of tea				
A	**576**	**38.9**	**23.9**	**49.7**
Or: Herb chicken	228	30.2	9.7	
Salad or steamed vegetables as above	80	2.2	1.2	8.0
Low-calorie soup	45	1.2	1.5	7.3
Cup of tea				
2 crackers	85	1.4	3.3	12.5
B	**438**	**35.0**	**15.7**	**27.8**

Total for day (*if no snacks*):

	K/CAL	PROTEIN (g)	FAT (g)	CBH (g)
TOTAL A	**1,234**	**79.1**	**45.9**	**142.7**
K/Calories (%)	1,300 (100%)	316.4 (24%)	413.1 (32%)	570.8
(44%)				
TOTAL B	**1,163**	**86.5**	**42.4**	**123.3**
K/Calories (%)	1,221 (100%)	346.0 (28%)	381.6 (31%)	493.2

BALANCED EATING PLAN NO.2: DAY'S MENU

	K/CAL	PROTEIN (g)	FAT (g)	CBH (g)
Breakfast				
Either: As for BEP no. 1				
A	**285**	**12.6**	**6.7**	**59.4**
Or: 1 medium bowl of sugar free cereal	65	2.1	0.6	13.6
1 cup skimmed milk	38	3.9	0.1	5.8
½ melon	34	0.6	0.3	8.1
Raspberries and strawberries	37	0.7	0.5	8.6
2 slices of toast (wholemeal) – dry	130	5.2	1.6	25.0
Cup of tea or coffee				
B	**304**	**12.5**	**3.1**	**61.1**
Lunch				
Either: As for BEP no. 1				
A	**373**	**27.6**	**15.3**	**33.6**
Or: Sliced chicken (no skin)	150	26.1	8.2	
Salad with lettuce, onions, tomato,				
½ banana	35	2.0	0.5	4.5
Low-fat dressing	60	0.1	6.6	3.0
1 slice toast (wholemeal) – dry	65	2.6	0.8	12.5
Cup of tea or coffee				
Freshly-squeezed orange juice (4oz)	57	0.8	0.2	14.6
B	**367**	**31.6**	**16.3**	**34.6**
Evening meal: Dinner				
Either: Vegetable-topped fish fillet	240	32.0	19.9	10.5
Waldorf special	80	2.2	1.2	8.0
1 slice calorie-reduced bread	40	1.3	0.4	6.6
½ teaspoon margarine	20		4.0	0.1
Cup of tea				
A	**380**	**35.5**	**25.5**	**25.2**
Or: Grilled fish and				
steamed broccoli	240	32.0	19.9	10.0
Boiled rice	171	3.2	0.3	39.0

No.2: Day's menu

	K/CAL	PROTEIN (g)	FAT (g)	CBH (g)
Evening meal: Dinner cont.				
1 slice toast (wholemeal) – dry	65	2.6	0.8	12.5
Cup of tea				
B	**476**	**37.8**	**21.0**	**61.5**
SNACK				
2 cups of microwave popcorn	104			16.2
A	**104**			**16.2**

Total for day

	K/CAL	PROTEIN (g)	FAT (g)	CBH (g)
TOTAL A	**1,142**	**75.7**	**47.5**	**134.4**
K/Calories (%)	1,268 (100%)	302.8 (24%)	427.5 (34%)	537.6 (42%)
TOTAL B	**1,147**	**81.9**	**40.4**	**157.2**
K/Calories (%)	1,320 (100%)	327.6 (24%)	383.6 (28%)	628.6 (48%)

However each meal can be interchanged so these totals are for guidance only

BALANCED EATING PLAN NO.3: DAY'S MENU

	K/CAL	PROTEIN (g)	FAT (g)	CBH (g)
Breakfast				
Either: As for BEP no. 1				
A	**285**	**12.6**	**6.7**	**59.4**
Or: ½ melon	34	0.6	0.3	8.1
2 slices of toast (wholemeal) – dry	130	5.2	1.6	25.0
2 eggs scrambled with peppers	148	6.6	12.4	1.8
Cup of tea or coffee				
B	**312**	**12.4**	**14.3**	**34.9**
Lunch				
Either: As for BEP no. 1				
A	**373**	**27.6**	**15.3**	**33.6**
Or: Salmon sandwich with	88	10.8	4.7	

No.3: Day's menu

	K/CAL	PROTEIN (g)	FAT (g)	CBH (g)
Lunch cont:				
tomato, lettuce, cucumber	35	2.0	0.5	4.5
2 slices wholemeal bread – dry	130	5.2	1.6	25.0
Pepper				
Cup of tea of coffee				
Freshly-squeezed orange juice (4oz)	57	0.8	0.2	14.6
B	**310**	**18.8**	**7.0**	**44.1**
Evening meal: Dinner				
Either: Cheesy macaroni	503	27.5	18.9	66.4
Salad	40	1.4	3.5	2.4
1 cup fresh young spinach leaves and				
5 fresh mushrooms – sliced				
Low-fat dressing	60	0.1	6.6	3.0
1 slice reduced-calorie bread	40	1.3	0.4	6.6
½ teaspoon low-calorie margarine	20		4.0	0.1
½ cup strawberries –				
sliced with low-fat yoghurt (4oz)	97	7.5	0.7	16.5
Cup of tea				
A	**760**	**37.8**	**34.1**	**95.0**
Or: Chicken or turkey salad	308	32.4	10.8	8.0
1 apple baked with lemon juice,				
honey, 2 dates and cinnamon	148	0.3	4.9	28.1
Cup of tea				
3 crackers – dry	127	2.6	5.0	18.1
B	**583**	**35.3**	**20.7**	**54.9**

Total for day

	K/CAL	PROTEIN (g)	FAT (g)	CBH (g)
TOTAL A	**1,418**	**78.0**	**56.1**	**188.0**
K/Calories (%)	1,569 (100%)	312.0 (20%)	504.9 (32%)	752.0 (48%)
TOTAL B	**1,205**	**66.5**	**42.0**	**133.9**
K/Calories (%)	1,180 (100%)	266.0 (23%)	378.0 (32%)	535.6 (45%)

However each meal can be interchanged so these totals are for guidance only

BALANCED EATING PLAN NO.4: DAY'S MENU

	K/CAL	Protein (g)	Fat (g)	CBH (g)
Breakfast				
Either: As for BEP no. 1				
A	**285**	**12.6**	**6.7**	**59.4**
Or: 1 egg omelette with mushrooms,				
tomato and onions	248	11.4	22.6	0.8
1 slice of toast (wholemeal) – dry	65	2.6	0.8	12.5
Cup of tea or coffee				
B	**313**	**14.0**	**23.4**	**13.3**
Lunch				
Either: As for BEP no. 1				
A	**373**	**27.6**	**15.3**	**33.6**
Or: Salad: 2 tomatoes, cucumber,				
peppers, mushrooms, parsley,				
lemon juice, lettuce	50	2.5	0.5	7.5
1 hard-boiled egg	72	5.6	5.2	0.3
Low-fat dressing	60	0.1	6.6	3.0
3 crackers – dry	127	2.6	5.0	18.8
Cup of tea or coffee				
B	**309**	**10.8**	**17.3**	**29.6**
Evening meal: Dinner				
Either: Lean sirloin steak – grilled, 3oz				
– topped with peppers and onions	305	24.5	22.4	
1 cup of green beans (steamed)	19	1.0	0.1	4.0
1 boiled small potato	72	1.8	0.1	17.1
Salad: lettuce leaf, ½ banana sliced,				
½ cup of raisins	80	2.2	1.2	12.5
Low-calorie mayonnaise	75	0.2	10.0	0.5
1 slice calorie-reduced bread	40	1.7	0.5	8.5
½ teaspoon low-calorie margarine	20		4.0	0.1
Cup of tea				
A	**611**	**31.4**	**38.3**	**42.7**

No.4: Day's menu

	K/CAL	PROTEIN (g)	FAT (g)	CBH (g)
Evening meal: Dinner cont.				
Or: Veal escalopes with fresh tomato, leek sauce, baked potato, spinach and tomato salad	400	34.2	21.4	30.2
Orange	59	1.2	0.3	14.4
Cup of tea				
2 crackers – dry	85	1.4	3.3	12.5
B	**544**	**36.8**	**25.0**	**57.1**

Total for day	K/CAL	PROTEIN (g)	FAT (g)	CBH (g)
TOTAL A	**1,269**	**71.6**	**60.3**	**135.7**
K/Calories (%)	1,372 (100%)	286.4 (20%)	542.7 (40%)	542.8 (40%)
TOTAL B	**1,166**	**61.6**	**65.7**	**100.0**
K/Calories (%)	1,238 (100%)	246.4 (20%)	591.3 (48%)	400.0 (32%)

However each meal can be interchanged so these totals are for guidance only

BALANCED EATING PLAN NO.5: DAY'S MENU

	K/CAL	PROTEIN (g)	FAT (g)	CBH (g)
Breakfast				
Either: As for BEP no. 1				
A	**285**	**12.6**	**6.7**	**59.4**
Or: ½ melon	34	0.6	0.3	8.1
1 bran muffin	170	2.9	3.2	22.1
Freshly-squeezed orange juice (4oz)	57	0.8	0.2	14.6
Cup of tea or coffee				
B	**261**	**4.3**	**3.7**	**44.8**
Lunch				
Either: As for BEP no. 1				
A	**373**	**27.6**	**15.3**	**33.6**

No.5: Day's menu

	K/CAL	Protein (g)	Fat (g)	CBH (g)
Lunch cont.				
Or: Tomato and tuna salad with lettuce, celery, apple, bean sprouts, hard-boiled egg	186	30.8	6.0	0.3
Low-fat dressing	60	0.1	6.6	3.0
2 crackers – dry	85	1.4	3.3	12.5
Cup of tea or coffee				
B	**331**	**32.3**	**15.9**	**15.8**
Evening meal: Dinner				
Either: Chick-pea bake	440	40.0	22.5	35.0
Baked potato (small)	164	2.0	9.1	19.7
2 tablespoons low-fat yoghurt	30	1.5	1.0	4.5
Salad: lettuce, celery, tomato, grated carrot	35	2.0	0.5	4.5
Low-calorie dressing	60	0.1	6.6	3.0
1 slice calorie-reduced bread	40	1.3	0.4	6.6
½ teaspoon low-calorie margarine	20		4.0	0.1
2 slices of pineapple – juice packed	59	0.5	0.1	15.8
Cup of tea				
A	**848**	**47.4**	**44.2**	**89.2**
Or: Pasta with steamed vegetables (no potato)	351	12.6	2.5	69.8
2 bread sticks	65	2.6	0.8	15.0
1 peach or pear	84	0.6	0.4	21.7
Cup of tea				
B	**500**	**15.8**	**3.7**	**106.5**

Total for day				
TOTAL A	**1,506**	**87.6**	**66.2**	**182.2**
K/Calories (%)	1,675 (100%)	350.4 (21%)	595.8 (35%)	728.8 (44%)
TOTAL B	**1,092**	**52.4**	**23.3**	**167.1**
K/Calories (%)	1,088 (100%)	209.6 (19%)	209.7 (19%)	668.4 (62%)

If BEP 'A' chosen then no other snacks for day. However each meal can be interchanged so these totals are for guidance only

BALANCED EATING PLAN NO.6: DAY'S MENU

	K/CAL	PROTEIN (g)	FAT (g)	CBH (g)
Breakfast				
Either: As for BEP no. 1				
A	285	12.6	6.7	59.4
Or: Fresh fruit salad (1 bowl)	210	2.8	1.0	52.8
1 slice of toast (wholemeal) – dry	65	5.2	1.6	25.0
Cup of tea or coffee				
B	275	8.0	2.6	77.8
Lunch				
Either: As for BEP no. 1				
A	373	27.6	15.3	33.6
Or: 4 shrimps (large)	220	43.4	2.8	1.2
lettuce, onions, cucumber, celery,				
tomato	35	2.0	0.5	4.5
Low-fat dressing	60	0.1	6.6	3.0
3 crackers – dry	127	2.6	5.0	18.8
Freshly-squeezed orange juice (4oz)	57	0.8	0.2	14.6
Cup of tea or coffee				
B	499	48.9	15.1	42.1
Evening meal: Dinner				
Either: 2 lean centre-cut pork chops,				
fat trimmed with steamed green beans				
(¾ cup)	696	34.8	60.8	
1 sweet potato	135	0.8	6.3	19.5
1 slice calorie-reduced bread	40	1.3	0.4	6.6
½ teaspoon low-calorie margarine	20		4.0	0.1
1 bowl of low-calorie soup	45	1.2	1.5	7.3
Cup of tea				
A	936	38.1	73.0	33.5
Or: Veal escalopes poached in herbs and				
lemon juice and chicken stock with				
4oz spaghetti	400	34.2	21.4	30.2

No.6: Day's menu

	K/CAL	PROTEIN (g)	FAT (g)	CBH (g)
Evening meal: Dinner cont.				
Asparagus	11	1.0	0.2	1.8
Green salad	50	2.5	0.5	7.5
2 breadsticks	65	2.6	0.8	15.0
Cup of tea				
B	**526**	**40.3**	**22.9**	**54.5**

Total for day

	K/CAL	PROTEIN (g)	FAT (g)	CBH (g)
TOTAL A	**1,594**	**78.3**	**95.0**	**126.5**
K/Calories (%)	1,674 (100%)	313.2 (19%)	855.0 (51%)	506.0 (30%)
TOTAL B	**1,300**	**97.2**	**40.6**	**174.4**
K/Calories (%)	1,452 (100%)	388.2 (27%)	365.4 (25%)	697.6 (48%)

If BEP 'A' chosen then no other snacks for day. However each meal can be interchanged so these totals are for guidance only

BALANCED EATING PLAN NO.7: DAY'S MENU

	K/CAL	PROTEIN (g)	FAT (g)	CBH (g)
Breakfast				
Either: As for BEP no. 1				
A	**285**	**12.6**	**6.7**	**59.4**
Or: 1 slice dry toast with	65	2.6	0.8	12.5
3 slices of smoked salmon, tomato,				
onion	88	10.8	4.7	
Freshly-squeezed orange juice (4oz)	57	0.8	0.2	14.6
Cup of tea or coffee				
B	**210**	**14.2**	**5.7**	**27.1**
Lunch				
Either: As for BEP no. 1				
A	**373**	**27.6**	**15.3**	**33.6**
Or: Turkey – 3 slices	309	33.0	18.5	

No.7: Day's menu

	K/CAL	PROTEIN (g)	FAT (g)	CBH (g)
Lunch cont.				
Salad: lettuce, celery, tomato	50	2.5	0.5	7.5
Hard-boiled egg	72	5.6	5.2	0.3
Low-fat dressing	60	0.1	6.6	3.0
2 crackers – dry	85	1.4	3.3	12.5
Freshly-squeezed orange juice (4oz)	57	0.8	0.2	14.6
Cup of tea or coffee				
B	**633**	**43.4**	**34.3**	**37.9**
Evening meal: Dinner				
Either: 8oz lasagne with low-fat cottage cheese and Italian sauce and 1 cup chopped broccoli (steamed)	410	12.9	3.2	75.1
2 slices calorie-reduced bread	80	2.6	0.8	13.2
1 teaspoon low-calorie margarine	40		8.0	0.2
Apple	53	0.3	0.3	13.8
Cup of tea				
A	**583**	**15.8**	**12.3**	**102.3**
Or: Steamed fish and cup of broccoli	240	32.0	19.9	10.0
Cup of rice boiled	171	3.2	0.3	39.0
Banana, berries in orange juice	145	2.3	1.3	35.2
2 crackers	85	1.4	3.3	12.5
Cup of tea				
B	**641**	**38.9**	**24.8**	**96.7**

Total for day

	K/CAL	PROTEIN (g)	FAT (g)	CBH (g)
TOTAL A	**1,241**	**56.0**	**34.3**	**195.3**
K/Calories (%)	1,314 (100%)	224.0 (17%)	308.7 (23%)	781.2 (60%)
TOTAL B	**1,484**	**96.5**	**64.8**	**161.7**
K/Calories (%)	1,616 (100%)	386.0 (24%)	583.2 (36%)	646.8 (40%)

If BEP 'A' chosen then no other snacks for day.

However each meal can be interchanged so these totals are for guidance only

Exchanges

To add variety of choice, we have also listed some possible 'exchanges'. An **'exchange'** refers to the alternatives or options in each of the nutritional categories. Exchanges are listed below. For example, one slice of bread can be exchanged for one medium (3oz or 90g) boiled, mashed or jacket potato. By using exchanges these diets can be altered to suit food preferences. You choose the foods you like, but keep to the restrictions we recommend. Use these exchanges to adapt our BEPs to your taste but it is important that you adhere closely to the daily allowances as only by doing this will you keep within the correct calorie balance between proteins, fats and carbohydrates.

Food group exchanges

Carbohydrate exchanges

♥ 1oz (30g) slice of bread, preferably wholemeal

♥ 1 medium 3oz (90g) boiled, mashed or jacket potato

♥ 2 crispbreads

♥ 3 tablespoons (2/3oz or 20g) unsweetened, preferably wholegrain, breakfast cereal – e.g. Sultana Bran, Raisin Splitz, Fruit 'n' Fibre or Oat Bran Flakes

♥ 1 Weetabix or 1 Shredded Wheat

♥ 4 tablespoons (5oz or 150g cooked weight) porridge made with water or milk from allowance

♥ 2 tablespoons (2oz or 60g cooked weight) rice or pasta – try the wholegrain variety

♥ 1 small (1oz or 30g) chapatti or pitta bread.

Protein exchanges

♥ 1oz (30g) lean meat – e.g. chicken, turkey and other poultry, beef, veal, lamb, mutton, pork, bacon, ham, tongue, rabbit and game, liver and kidney. Well-grilled lean beefburgers and low-fat sausages occasionally

♥ 2oz (60g) white fish, e.g. cod, haddock, plaice, whiting, lemon sole

♥ 2oz (60g) shellfish, e.g. prawns, crabs, lobster

♥ 1oz (30g) oily fish, e.g. herring, kipper, mackerel, salmon, tuna, sardines

♥ ¾ oz (23g) cheese, e.g. edam, reduced fat cheddar cheese

♥ 2oz (60g) cottage cheese or quark

♥ 3.5oz (105g) baked beans or 2.5oz (75g) haricot, kidney or butter beans, or lentils (cooked weight)

♥ 1 egg (no more than 4 per week).

Fat exchanges

♥ ½ oz (15g) poly-unsaturated margarine

♥ 1oz (30g) low-fat spread

♥ 1 tablespoon (15ml) poly-unsaturated cooking oil, or 1 tablespoon (15ml) mono-unsaturated cooking oil.

Note: ¼ oz margarine or ½ oz low-fat spread can be exchanged for 1 tablespoon low-calorie mayonnaise/dressing.

Milk exchanges

♥ ⅔ pt (400ml) semi skimmed

♥ 1 pt (600ml) skimmed.

Note: One 150g pot of low-fat natural or diet yoghurt can be taken instead of ⅓ pt semi-skimmed or ½ pt skimmed milk.

Fruit exchanges

♥ 1 medium apple, orange, pear, peach, nectarine or small banana

♥ 2 tangerines/satsumas, 4oz (120g) cherries, 2 damsons/greengages, 3oz (90g) grapes, 4oz (120g) pineapple or up to 6oz (180g) strawberries, raspberries, blackberries or redcurrants, or 3oz (90g) fresh mango

♥ 1oz (30g) dried fruit – e.g. sultanas, figs, apricots, prunes, etc.

♥ 1 portion (4oz or 120g) fruit tinned in natural juice

> *Not all the changes may be necessary to convert your current diet into one that's nutrionally balanced...*

Until you are familiar with portion size and the calorie value of those portions, weigh your food

♥ 1 small glass (¼ pt or 150ml) unsweetened fruit juice

♥ 1 portion (4oz or 120g) stewed fruit without sugar – an artificial sweetener may be used but should be added after cooking.

Foods allowed freely

Remember, no butter, dressing or other fatty complements, but you may eat unlimited amounts of these foods in addition to your calorie-controlled diet.

Vegetables and salad

Artichoke, asparagus, aubergine, french and runner beans, beansprouts, beetroot, broad beans, broccoli, brussel sprouts, cabbage, carrots, cauliflower, celeriac, celery, chicory, cucumber, endive, leeks, lettuce, marrow, mushrooms, mustard and cress, okra, onions, parsley, parsnips, peas, red and green peppers, radishes, spinach, sweetcorn, swedes, tomatoes, turnips and watercress.

Fruit

Gooseberries, grapefruit, lemons, loganberries, melon and fresh currants.

Seasonings

Pepper, mustard, vinegar, worcester sauce, herbs, spices, stock cubes, gelatine and tomato purée.

Drinks

Water, soda water, tea, coffee, low-calorie squashes and fizzy drinks, e.g. Diet Pepsi, Diet Lilt, One Cal.

Sweetening agents

Any tablet, granulated or liquid artificial sweetener, e.g. Canderel, Sweetex and Hermasetas.

Foods allowed in moderation

Jam, honey, marmalade, sweet pickle, chutney, fat-free salad dressing and fat-free mayonnaise.

Foods not allowed at all

You will have a detrimental effect on your weight loss if you consume these items – *keep away from them!*

Sweet/sugary foods

Sugar, glucose, dextrose, sorbitol (the sweetener used in some diabetic products), syrup, treacle, lemon curd, sweets, chocolate (including diabetic sweets and chocolates), jelly, ice cream, tinned fruit in syrup, mousse, instant desserts and bottled sauces.

Fatty foods

All fried foods and visibly fatty foods, e.g. fatty meats, cooking oils, lards, dripping or fats of any kind (margarine or low-fat spread only as allowed). Sweet biscuits, cakes, pastry, puddings, thickened savoury and sweet sauces, custard, sausage rolls, meat pies and dumplings. Cream, cream substitutes, evaporated and condensed milk, cream cheese, salad cream/dressing, mayonnaise and sandwich spread. Salads with a dressing, e.g. coleslaw, potato salad. Cream sauces, chips, crisps, nuts and avocado pear.

Drinks

Alcohol in any form – wines, beers, ciders, etc. Sweetened fizzy drinks, sweetened fruit squash cordials, malted and bedtime drinks, bottled coffee, instant lemon tea, coffee and tea whiteners.

Daily calorie tracers

We would also recommend that, until you are familiar with portion size and the calorie value of those portions, you weigh your food. This will help greatly when you eat out with friends or at restaurants, where it is impossible to weigh food, but your judgement of the size of servings will have been developed by your 'home training'. One of the most important aspects of the nutrition plan is the calorie tracer. Every day for a few weeks you should fill in your tracer. It is the most effective way of monitoring your progress and

READY RECKONER OF FOOD VALUES

STANDARD MEASURES

♥ 1 CUP   8 FLUID OUNCES

♥ 1 TABLESPOON   20 ML

♥ 1 TEASPOON   5 ML

NOTE: The values below are computed in grams, the ounce column is only approximate.

FOODS	WEIGHT ounces	WEIGHT grams	DESCRIPTIVE MEASURE (approximate)	PROTEIN g	FAT g	CARBO-HYDRATE g	K/cal
Bread							
Brown	$\frac{7}{8}$	25	1 slice (4 x $3\frac{1}{2}$ x $\frac{1}{3}$ inches)	2.0	0.5	12.3	60
	$1\frac{1}{4}$	50	2 slices	4.0	0.9	24.6	121
Brown + 4% skim	$\frac{7}{8}$	26	1 slice (4 x $3\frac{1}{2}$ x $\frac{1}{3}$ inches)	2.2	0.6	12.1	62
milk powder	$1\frac{1}{4}$	52	2 slices	4.4	1.2	24.1	124
Rye, light	$\frac{3}{4}$	22	1 slice (4 x $2\frac{3}{4}$ x $\frac{1}{3}$ inches)	1.7	0.4	10.8	53
	$1\frac{1}{2}$	44	2 slices	3.3	0.7	21.6	105
Rye, dark	$1\frac{1}{8}$	32	1 slice ($4\frac{1}{2}$ x $3\frac{1}{2}$ x $\frac{3}{8}$ inches)	2.5	0.5	15.6	76
	$2\frac{1}{4}$	64	2 slices	4.9	1.0	31.2	152
Raisin	$\frac{7}{8}$	26	1 slice (4 x $3\frac{1}{4}$ x $\frac{3}{8}$ inches)	1.7	0.8	13.5	67
	$1\frac{3}{4}$	52	2 slices	3.3	1.5	27.0	133
White	$\frac{7}{8}$	23	1 slice (4 x 4 x $\frac{1}{3}$ inches)	1.8	0.4	11.5	56
	$1\frac{5}{8}$	46	2 slices	3.6	0.7	23.0	112
White + 4% skim	$\frac{7}{8}$	24	1 slice (4 x 4 x $\frac{1}{3}$ inches)	2.0	0.6	11.6	59
milk powder	$1\frac{5}{8}$	48	2 slices	4.0	1.2	23.2	118
White, starch reduced	$\frac{5}{8}$	18	1 slice ($3\frac{1}{2}$ x $3\frac{1}{2}$ x $\frac{1}{3}$ inches)	1.7	0.5	8.5	44
	$1\frac{1}{4}$	36	2 slices	3.4	0.9	17.0	88
Wholemeal	$1\frac{1}{8}$	32	1 slice ($4\frac{1}{4}$ x 4 x $\frac{1}{3}$ inches)	2.6	0.8	15.0	74
	$2\frac{1}{4}$	64	2 slices	5.2	1.5	29.9	147
Breakfast cereal							
Cornflakes	$\frac{1}{2}$	14	$\frac{1}{2}$ cup	1.2	Tr	11.8	50
	1	27	1 cup	2.3	0.1	23.6	100
Oatmeal, cooked (1:3)	4	117	$\frac{1}{2}$ cup	2.4	1.3	11.7	65
	8	234	1 cup	4.7	2.6	23.4	129
Rice bubbles	$\frac{1}{2}$	13	$\frac{1}{2}$ cup	0.8	0.1	11.7	51
	$\frac{7}{8}$	26	1 cup	1.5	0.2	23.4	101

FOODS	WEIGHT ounces	WEIGHT grams	DESCRIPTIVE MEASURE (approximate)	PROTEIN g	FAT g	CARBO-HYDRATE g	K/cal
Wheatflake biscuit	5⁄8	17	1 biscuit	2.1	0.2	12.2	60
	1 1⁄8	33	2 biscuits	4.2	0.4	24.4	120
Biscuits, savoury and sweet							
Salada	3⁄8	12	3 biscuits	1.3	0.9	8.8	48
Sao	3⁄8	9	1 biscuit	0.7	1.7	6.3	43
	5⁄8	18	2 biscuits	1.4	3.3	12.5	85
Ryvita	3⁄8	10	1 biscuit	1.0	0.3	7.5	34
	5⁄8	19	2 biscuits	1.9	0.5	15.0	68
Vita wheat	1⁄4	6	1 biscuit	0.5	0.6	4.2	23
	3⁄8	11	2 biscuits	1.0	1.2	8.3	46
Wheatmeal	1⁄4	8	1 biscuit	0.6	1.0	6.2	35
Cream filled assorted	5⁄8	19	1 biscuit	0.9	4.8	12.8	95
Chocolate coated, plain	3⁄4	20	2 biscuits	1.2	2.9	15.0	87
Plain, sweet	5⁄8	16	2 biscuits	1.0	2.0	12.3	68
Flour							
Plain	3⁄8	10	1 tablespoon	1.1	0.2	7.4	36
	3⁄4	20	2 tablespoons	2.2	0.4	14.8	72
	1	28	1⁄4 cup	3.1	0.5	20.7	101
	2	56	1⁄2 cup	6.2	1.0	41.4	202
	4	112	1 cup	12.4	2.0	82.8	403
Eggs							
Egg, whole, medium	1 1⁄2	45	one	5.6	5.2	0.3	72
	3 1⁄8	90	two	11.2	10.4	0.6	144
Egg, white, medium	1	28	one	2.9	Tr	0.2	14
Egg, yolk, medium	5⁄8	17	one	2.8	5.2	0.1	59
Butter							
		5	1 teaspoon	Tr	3.8	Tr	34
	5⁄8	19	1 tablespoon	0.1	15.4	0.1	138
	1 3⁄8	38	2 tablespoons	0.2	30.8	0.2	276
	8	228	1⁄2 lb packet	1.8	185.4	1.6	1,658
	16	456	1 lb packet	3.6	370.7	3.2	3,315

FOODS	WEIGHT ounces	WEIGHT grams	DESCRIPTIVE MEASURE (approximate)	PROTEIN g	FAT g	CARBO- HYDRATE g	K/cal
Fish							
baked or steamed, no fat	3½	100	2 small fillets	19.4	1.7	0	95
crumbed and fried	3½	100	1 fillet	18.4	14.4	11.6	253
fried in batter	3½	100	1 fillet	19.2	13.1	14.3	249
Fruits							
fresh:							
Apple	3½	100	1 small	0.3	0.3	13.8	53
Apricot	3½	100	3 medium	0.8	0.2	11.4	45
Banana	3½	100	1 medium – 6 inches long	1.1	0.3	22.5	87
Grapefruit	4¼	120	½ (4 inches diameter)	0.6	0.2	11.0	44
Grapes	3½	100	20–22	0.7	0.4	16.8	66
Mandarins	3½	100	1 large or 2 small	0.8	0.3	11.2	46
Oranges	4½	130	1 medium (2¾ inches diameter)	1.2	0.3	14.4	59
Passionfruit	1	30	1 medium	0.7	0.2	6.3	27
Peaches	3¾	110	1 medium (2½ inches diameter)	0.7	0.1	11.7	45
Pear	5¼	150	1 medium	0.6	0.4	21.7	84
Pineapple	2¾	80	1 slice (3½ x 3½ x ½ inches)	0.4	0.2	10.8	42
Tomato	3¾	110	1 medium	1.1	0.3	4.5	23
dried:							
Currants	⅜	11	1 tablespoon	0.2	Tr	8.0	30
Raisins	½	13	1 tablespoon	0.2	Tr	9.7	36
Sultanas	½	13	1 tablespoon	0.2	Tr	9.9	37
Dates	1⅛	33	5 to 6 pitted	0.7	0.2	25.3	95
Juices, canned and sweetened							
Apple	4¼	120	½ cup	0.1	Tr	13.8	50
Grape	4¼	120	½ cup	0.2	Tr	19.9	79
Grapefruit	4¼	120	½ cup	0.6	0.1	15.3	57
Orange	4¼	120	½ cup	0.8	0.2	14.6	57
Pineapple	4¼	120	½ cup	0.5	0.1	15.8	59
Tomato	4¼	120	½ cup	1.2	0.2	4.9	24

FOODS	WEIGHT ounces	WEIGHT grams	DESCRIPTIVE MEASURE (approximate)	PROTEIN g	FAT g	CARBO-HYDRATE g	K/cal
Meats							
Beef							
fillet steak, average, grilled	4½	130	2 average	31.8	39.5	0	493
fillet steak, lean, grilled	5	140	2 average	39.6	12.3	0	280
T-bone, average, grilled	3½	100	1 average (no bone)	24.5	22.4	0	305
T-bone, lean, grilled	3¾	110	1 average (no bone)	31.1	9.6	0	220
Hamburger with cereal	2⅝	75	1 patty	11.4	14.8	11.9	223
Roast topside, lean	2⅝	75	1 slice (3 x 3 x ½ inches)	20.1	11.3	0	188
Sausage, thick, grilled	3¾	110	2 average (3½ x 1¼ inches)	16.7	24.3	10.5	339
Chicken							
boiled	4	115	1 breast	30.2	9.7	0	228
fried	4¾	135	1 breast	38.6	17.7	3.9	342
Lamb							
average chop, grilled	3¾	110	2 average (no bone)	20.4	33.7	0	391
chop, lean, grilled	3½	100	2 average (no bone)	25.5	8.1	0	181
roast, leg	2⅝	75	2 slices (3 x 3 x ¼ inches)	14.8	23.1	0	267
Veal							
cutlet, crumbed and fried	5	140	2 average (no bone)	27.7	25.6	12.1	400
cutlet, grilled	3½	100	2 average (no bone)	30.7	13.0	0	247
roast, rump	2⅝	75	2 slices (3¼ x 2¼ x ¼ inches)	20.8	8.8	0	168
Pork							
chop, grilled	2¾	80	1 chop	17.4	30.4	0	348
roast, leg	2⅝	75	2 slices (5½ x 3¾ x ⅛ inches)	15.0	33.6	0	367
Bacon							
raw	1⅜	40	1 strip 13 inches long	4.1	23.6	0.4	231
fried	¾	21	1 strip (40g raw weight)	4.1	13.4	0.4	142
grilled	½	15	1 strip (40g raw weight)	4.1	8.9	0.4	99
Sausage meats							
Devon	1¾	50	2 slices (4 x 4 x ⅛ inches)	7.3	9.2	1.9	120
Frankfurter, boiled	3½	100	2 average (3 x 1¼ inches diameter)	13.0	23.8	2.0	280
Dairy							
Milk	¾	20	1 tablespoon	0.7	0.8	0.9	13
fresh	2	58	¼ cup	1.9	2.2	2.6	39
	4	115	½ cup	3.8	4.4	5.2	77

FOODS	WEIGHT ounces	WEIGHT grams	DESCRIPTIVE MEASURE (approximate)	PROTEIN g	FAT g	CARBO-HYDRATE g	K/cal
Milk, fresh	8	230	1 cup	7.6	8.7	10.5	154
	5	142	¼ pint	4.7	5.4	6.6	96
	10	284	½ pint	9.4	10.8	13.1	191
	6¾	190	⅓ pint	6.3	7.2	8.7	127
	20	570	1 pint	18.8	21.6	26.2	382
	40	1,140	1 quart	37.6	43.2	52.4	764
Milk, skimmed	¾	20	1 tablespoon	0.7	Tr	1.0	7
	2	58	¼ cup	2.0	Tr	2.8	20
	4	115	½ cup	3.9	0.1	5.5	40
	8	230	1 cup	7.8	0.2	11.0	80
	20	570	1 pint	19.3	0.6	27.3	199
Milk, full cream, dried			1 teaspoon	0.7	0.6	0.8	12
	⅜	9	1 tablespoon	2.6	2.4	3.3	46
	⅞	25	¼ cup	7.0	6.5	8.9	126
	1¾	49	½ cup	14.0	13.0	17.9	253
	3½	98	1 cup	27.9	25.9	35.8	505
Milk, skimmed, dried			1 teaspoon	1.0	Tr	1.3	10
	⅜	11	1 tablespoon	4.2	0.1	5.5	41
	2	56	½ cup	21.6	0.6	28.1	209
	4	112	1 cup	43.1	1.1	56.2	418
Cream	⅔	20	1 tablespoon	0.4	7.6	0.6	73
	1⅜	40	2 tablespoons	0.8	15.2	1.2	146
	2	60	¼ cup	1.3	22.8	1.8	218
	4¼	120	½ cup	2.5	45.6	3.6	437
	6¾	190	⅓ pint	3.9	72.2	5.7	692
	10	284	½ pint	6.0	107.9	8.5	1,034
Milk, condensed	⅞	27	1 tablespoon	2.5	2.5	14.7	93
	1⅞	54	2 tablespoons	5.0	5.0	29.4	186
	2⅝	75	¼ cup	6.8	6.8	40.7	259
	5¼	150	½ cup	13.6	13.6	81.4	517
	14	398	1 tin (14oz)	36.0	36.0	217.0	1,376
Milk, evaporated	¾	21	1 tablespoon	1.7	1.7	2.2	32
	2¼	63	¼ cup	5.0	5.1	6.5	94
	4⅜	125	½ cup	9.9	10.1	13.0	188
	14½	412	1 tin (14½oz)	32.5	33.4	42.8	618

FOODS	WEIGHT ounces	WEIGHT grams	DESCRIPTIVE MEASURE (approximate)	PROTEIN g	FAT g	CARBO-HYDRATE g	K/cal
Cheese							
cheddar cheese	¾	20	1 inch cube	5.2	6.6	0	80
packet cheese	¾	21	1 slice (3¾ x 3½ x ⅛ inches)	4.6	5.3	0.2	67
grated cheese	⅜	9	1 tablespoon	3.7	2.9	0	41
processed cheese spread	⅝	19	1 tablespoon	4.0	5.1	0.2	63
cream cheese	⅝	19	1 tablespoon	1.7	6.1	0.6	66
cottage cheese, creamed	¾	20	1 tablespoon	2.7	0.8	0.6	21
Yoghurt							
flavoured and fruit	8	230	1 carton	9.8	8.0	25.0	214
plain	8	230	1 carton	10.1	8.2	13.1	165
low-fat	8	230	1 carton	13.5	0.2	15.8	119
Sugar							
	⅛	4	1 teaspoon	0	0	4.0	16
	⅝	16	1 tablespoon	0	0	16.0	62
	1¾	50	¼cup	0	0	50.0	195
	3½	100	½ cup	0	0	99.9	390
Vegetables							
Asparagus	2	60	3 medium spears	1.0	0.2	1.8	11
Beans, boiled	2	60	½ cup	1.0	0.1	4.0	19
Beetroot, canned	1	30	2 slices	0.3	Tr	2.3	10
Carrot, raw	2	60	1 small 4 inches long	0.5	0.1	5.1	22
Cauliflower, boiled	2	60	½ cup flower pieces	1.3	0.1	2.5	14
Mushroom, sautéed in butter	2	60	6 to 7 small ones	1.4	6.3	2.4	66
Peas, boiled	2	56	⅓ cup	3.0	0.2	7.6	39
Peanuts	1⅓	43	1 small packet	11.3	20.9	8.3	249
Pumpkin, boiled	2	60	¼ cup mashed	0.6	0.1	4.2	19
Spinach, boiled	2	60	⅓ cup	1.6	0.2	2.4	15
Potato, mashed	¾	20	1 tablespoon	0.4	0.1	2.6	13
crisps	1	28	1 packet	1.2	8.8	11.0	125
boiled	3⅛	90	1 medium	1.8	0.1	17.1	72
baked	3⅛	90	1 medium	2.0	9.1	19.7	164
french-fried	3⅛	90	17 to 18 pieces 2 inches long	3.4	12.7	29.3	241

educating yourself to assess foods readily for future guidance. It is also an enormous assistance in controlling your 'snack impulses' – if you eat, you have to write it down. As you record your calorie intake you begin to quickly learn the calorie value of various foods and the proportions of carbohydrate, fat and protein in them. You will soon be able to see exactly where you need to change your eating habits.

In summary

To finish, let us remind you of points to watch in order to ensure you make the right start:

♥ **Eating out at restaurants can pose potential problems**. Remember that you are always in control of the food you order. For a starter try melon, or soup – preferably tomato based or a salad with the dressing on the side so that you can add to taste, not to excess. For main course try pasta with tomato sauce (not cream or oil), or grilled fish, chicken or meat with steamed vegetables and jacket or boiled potatoes (no butter).

♥ **If you are not going out for lunch why not prepare sandwiches or a bean salad at home and bring it to work**. If you go to a sandwich bar, order a wholemeal roll with turkey, ham or chicken. **You should ask for no butter**. Try mustard, or pickle instead if you do need a garnish. Consider a baked potato with baked beans, again no butter. Always remember the principles of good nutrition when you order.

♥ **Food shopping** – 'shop right to eat right'. Do not go shopping hungry and buy enough fruit and vegetables to last you for the week to come.

♥ **Eat plenty of complex carbohydrates** – they will keep you full while you lose weight.

♥ **Reduce the amount of fat, fatty foods and sugar** you eat and the **alcohol** that you drink.

♥ **Do not add salt** to cooking or to cooked food at the table.

We have supplied you with all the tools you need throughout the programme but it is YOU who needs to take control.

The programme is a learning process that will help you to change your eating habits for life.

Best of luck, work hard, and you cannot fail to lose at least ten to sixteen pounds during the first six weeks of the programme. Thousands have at our club in London and the few who did not achieve this figure were only those who found the discipline too much for 42 days. It is not that long a time, the sacrifice is well worth it and it is not as if we are asking you to live like a monk – just to practise some self control for a few weeks. I suppose the course is really a test of character as well.

Tricks of the grocery trade

It is important to learn how to use the compulsory information on the packaging of all foodstuffs listing contents and nutrients.

Follow these rules:

1 Complex rather than simple carbohydrates are much the healthier choice. Go for products which break their carbohydrate content down (you can be sure that if they don't it is not good news).

2 Check the actual contents of the pack against the contents listed. Usually the label is restricted to an analysis of a 100g serving of the product but, at a glance, this is often taken to be the analysis of the package itself, which in reality could contain three to four times the calories listed.

3 Some packages go even further and show the nutrient analysis of a 30g 'serving'. No one eats only 30g of anything except a spread or dressing. This is just over 1oz in nutrient terms. Have in mind your normal serving size, and also be familiar with gram and ounce ratios.

One of the most important aspects of the nutrition plan is the calorie tracer

> *Grams don't really count except as a basis for your sums*

4 Remember the 4–9–4 rule, i.e. there are four calories in every gram of protein and carbohydrate but nine in every gram of fat. So when you see the grams of protein, fat and carbohydrate, these should be multiplied out to check the actual percentages of these three major nutrients in the total calories.

The food manufacturers do not do this for you. Rather, they show the total number of calories, then switch to grams, usually making up a 100g total so that the percentage of the total looks easy.

Wrong. The fat percentage of total calories is more than twice this. You should practise doing these calculations in order to keep track of precisely the amount of each nutrient you are consuming on a day to day basis.

Let's take a popular cereal: **Kellogg's Nut Corn Flakes.** The analysis on the side of the packet shows, per 100g (remember a medium size packet itself is 500g):

Calories	390
Protein	7g
Fat	3.5g
Carbohydrate	82g
(Sugar – simple	35g)
(Starch – complex	47g)

But converting this information to calories and percentage terms, it is:

Calories	390 – 100%
Protein	28 – 7%
Fat	32 – 8%
Carbohydrate	330 – 85%

Without adding fresh fruit this is a quick fix, short-term breakfast, almost in the same category as a chocolate bar or cola drink in actual nutritional value (and this is without any milk).

Another example, **Bran Muesli:**

100g	357	calories	100%
Protein	10.6	42	12%
Fat	6.1	55	15%
Carbohydrate	64.8	260	73%
(simple	23.9)		
(complex	30.9)		

This is much better nutritionally, especially if taken with skimmed milk and fresh fruit.

Far be it from us to comment upon the famous 'slimmers' breakfast' of Kellogg's Special K, but, if you believe the propaganda, I beg you – do some analysing of your own. There are many healthier, more economical, and far more effective breakfast products for slimmers around.

In summary, remember the traps when shopping. Check those labels, apply the multiples and see what you are getting with regard to the correct nutritional 20–30–50, protein–fat–carbohydrate formula, and the total calorie content, of each serving. Grams don't really count except as a basis for your sums and a 30g serving is nonsense for most products; we all take much larger helpings than that.

Food tolerances and allergies

There are certain foods, some of which we like, others which our instincts warn us about, that have disastrous physiological effects when they are consumed. Bilious attacks, diarrhoea, rashes, acute abdominal swelling and pains can occur. Food allergies are a part of your genetic make-up and stay with you for life. Once identified, usually by trial and error, you have no option but to ban them from your menus for ever. Fortunately, there are usually very few foods which fit into this category.

Recently, a laboratory in the UK has developed a 'Nu Tron' test which is designed to identify food tolerances and intolerances. These are identified at the laboratory by exposing blood samples, gained from individuals, to 92 different foods and checking the reaction within the block enzymes.

The theory is that a list of intolerant foods can be produced which your digestion finds hard to absorb – especially those with a high fat content which is transferred to the body tissues where it adds to the body's fat storage and increases fluid retention.

Unlike those foods to which your body is allergic, the range of the tolerant/intolerant foods can change over the years and you should go and be re-tested every five years, or so.

If the body tolerant foods are incorporated into your BEP, the gut loses this permeability, thus digesting and excreting the fats normally without passing a high percentage through to the blood system and on to the tissues. In short, *you'll lose weight quite quickly in the short term* and, then, whilst continuing to follow the system, *maintain this loss*. Of course, calories still have to be balanced, as do nutrients, but the concept appears to work and to have a credible biological basis.

Combining Foods

A growing school of thought is supporting a concept in which foods of different nutritional elements should not be eaten at the same meal. The diagram above summarizes this theory succinctly.

The rules for combining foods were first developed more than 70 years ago by a famous American scientist, Dr William Howard Hay. His books, *A New Health Era* and *Health Via Food*, spell out his theories on keeping food intake simple but understanding the reaction certain types of food have upon each other.

Both books were widely acclaimed and extremely controversial but the Hay formula is still widely recommended by nutritionists. The Hay system is based on the importance of balancing blood chemistry. Everything we eat is either *acid forming* or *alkaline forming*. Dr Hay analysed what foods do which and formulated the rule that, although such foods should be balanced in a day's eating plan, you should avoid

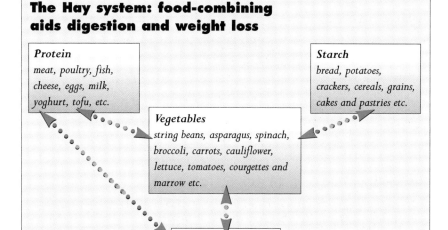

The Hay system: food-combining aids digestion and weight loss

Protein
meat, poultry, fish, cheese, eggs, milk, yoghurt, tofu, etc.

Starch
bread, potatoes, crackers, cereals, grains, cakes and pastries etc.

Vegetables
string beans, asparagus, spinach, broccoli, carrots, cauliflower, lettuce, tomatoes, courgettes and marrow etc.

Fruits
one type at a time: do not mix fruits

The Hay system rules are relatively simple:

1 Starches and sugars should not be taken with proteins and acid fruits at the same meal

2 Vegetables, salads and fruits should form the major part of the diet

3 Proteins, starches and fats should be taken in small amounts

4 Only wholegrain and unprocessed starches should be eaten and all refined processed foods should be taboo – particularly white flour, sugar and all foods made with them as well as highly processed fats such as margarine (butter is better)

5 An interval of at least four hours should elapse between meals of different character, especially following meals including protein.

Dr Hay recommended that changes to anybody's habits should be adopted slowly and that, if you wish to discover for yourself the effect of his teachings, try just rules 1 and 2 at first and slowly learn to incorporate the remainder over an eight-week period.

mixing them at any one sitting. The following charts illustrate the way these types of diets are formulated.

Dr Hay himself was an interesting man. Born in Hartstorm, Pennsylvania, US, in 1866, he grew up dedicated to medicine and, after graduating from the University of New York in March 1891, he went on to spend the next 16 years of his life practising medicine until he became very ill with high blood pressure (he

TABLE OF COMPATIBLE FOODS

◀ **can be combined** ▶   ◀ **can be combined** ▶

Columns I and III are incompatible	*Can be combined with either Col. I or Col. III*	*Columns I and III are incompatible*
I FOR PROTEIN MEALS	II NEUTRAL FOODS	III FOR STARCH MEALS

I FOR PROTEIN MEALS	II NEUTRAL FOODS	III FOR STARCH MEALS
Proteins	**Nuts**	**Cereals**
Meat of all kinds:	All except peanuts	Wholegrain: wheat, barley, maize
Beef, lamb, pork, venison		(corn), oats, millet, rice (brown,
Poultry: chicken, duck, goose, turkey	**Fats**	unpolished), rye
Game: pheasant, partridge, grouse, hare	Butter	Bread 100% wholewheat
Fish of all kinds including shellfish	Cream	Flour 100% or 85%
Milk, including soya	Egg yolks	Oatmeal – medium
(combines best with fruit and should not	Olive oil (virgin)	
be served at a meat meal)	Sunflower seed oil	
Yoghurt, including soya	Sesame seed oil (cold pressed)	
Fruits	**Vegetables**	**Sweet fruits**
Apples	All green and root vegetables except	Bananas – ripe
Apricots (fresh and dried)	potatoes and Jerusalem artichokes	Custard apples
Blackberries	Asparagus	Dates
Blueberries	Aubergines (eggplants)	Figs (fresh and dried)
Cherries	Beans (all fresh green beans)	Grapes – extra sweet
Currants (black, red or white if ripe)	Beetroot	Papaya (paw paw) if *very* ripe
Gooseberries (if ripe)	Broccoli	Pears if *very* sweet and ripe
Grapefruit	Brussels sprouts	Currants
Grapes	Cabbage	Raisins
Guavas	Calabrese	Sultanas
Kiwis	Carrots	
Lemons	Cauliflower	**Vegetables**
Limes	Celery	Jerusalem artichokes
Loganberries	Celeriac	Potatoes
Lychees	Kohlrabi	Pumpkin
Mangoes (best eaten *alone* as fruit meal)	Leeks	Sweet potatoes

◄ **can be combined** ►   ◄ **can be combined** ►

Columns I and III are incompatible	*Can be combined with either Col. I or Col. III*	*Columns I and III are incompatible*
I FOR PROTEIN MEALS	II NEUTRAL FOODS	III FOR STARCH MEALS

I FOR PROTEIN MEALS

Fruits (cont.)
Nectarines
Oranges
Passion fruit
Pears
Pineapples
Prunes (for occasional use)
Raspberries
Satsumas
Strawberries
Tangerines
N.B. Cranberries, plums
and rhubarb are not recommended

Salad dressings
Fresh dressing made with oil and lemon
juice or cider vinegar
Cream dressing
Mayonnaise (homemade)

II NEUTRAL FOODS

Vegetables (cont.)
Marrow
Mushrooms
Onions
Parsnips
Peas
Spinach
Swedes
Turnips

Saladings

Avocados   Sweetcorn
Chicory (endive)   Tomatoes
Cucumber   (uncooked)
Fennel   Watercress
Garlic
Lettuce   *Herbs and*
Mustard and cress   *flavourings*
Peppers   Chives
(red and green)   Mint
Radishes   Parsley
Spring onions   Sage
Sprouted legumes   Tarragon
Sprouted seeds   Thyme

III FOR STARCH MEALS

Milk and yoghurt
only in moderation

Salad dressings
Sweet or soured cream
Olive oil or cold pressed seed oils
Fresh tomato juice with oil and seasoning

TABLE OF COMPATIBLE FOODS

◀ **can be combined** ▶   ◀ **can be combined** ▶

Columns I and III are incompatible	*Can be combined* *with either Col. I or Col. III*	*Columns I and III are incompatible*
I FOR PROTEIN MEALS	II NEUTRAL FOODS	III FOR STARCH MEALS

◆ *Use only organically grown fruit*
◆◆ *All soya products are processed;*
   use sparingly

I FOR PROTEIN MEALS	II NEUTRAL FOODS	III FOR STARCH MEALS
	Herbs and flavourings (cont.)	
	◆ Grated lemon rind	
	◆ Grated orange rind	
	Seeds and seed spreads	
	Sunflower	
	Sesame	
	Pumpkin	
	Bran	
	Wheat or oat bran	
	Wheatgerm or oatgerm	
Sugar substitute	*Sugar substitute*	*Sugars*
Diluted frozen orange juice	Raisins and grape juice	Barbados sugar
Concentrated apple juice	Honey	Honey – in strict moderation
	Maple syrup	
For vegetarians		
(but not recommended)		
Legumes		
Lentils		
◆◆ Soya beans		
Kidney beans		
Chick peas		
Butter beans		
Pinto beans		
◆◆ Tofu		
Alcohol	*Alcohol*	*Alcohol*
Dry red and white wines	Whisky	Lager
Dry cider	Gin	Beer

was grossly overweight), Bright's disease and, finally, a dilated heart for which there was no permanent cure in those days. Seemingly, his career and his life were over at the relatively young age of 41.

After being warned by his doctors to 'put his affairs in order', he became inspired to try another way and began to 'eat fundamentally'. Within three months he had reversed all the trends, reduced his weight by about 3½ stone (50 lbs) to 12 st 7 lbs (175 lbs). He had begun to exercise regularly and was soon running quite long distances.

He resumed his medical career and, for the next four years, concentrated on treating his patients along dietary lines to either prove or disprove his theory that 'we are what we eat'.

To get it right, Dr Hay never claimed his diets or eating plans could cure any diseases, not even his own. *His contention was that nature cures but by eating the correct foods in the right way, you allow nature a full hand to do her work.*

His message was that there is one underlying cause of all the common diseases – wrong chemical conditions in the body. This chemical imbalance comes about from the manufacture and accumulation of acid end-products of digestion and metabolism in amounts greater than the body can eliminate.

The result – a lowering of the body's natural alkaline reserve leading to a departure from health which, if not actually promoting disease, provides a fertile base for its development.

'The science of medicine,' wrote Dr Hay, 'takes no cognisance of this accumulation until disease has developed.'

At that time, Dr Hay's statements were medical heresy as the profession was still completely committed to *treatment* rather than *prevention*.

Dr Hay lived on until 1940 preaching his doctrine. Sadly, just as he died after a serious accident, general medical opinion began to appreciate the important relationship between nutrition and health. He was

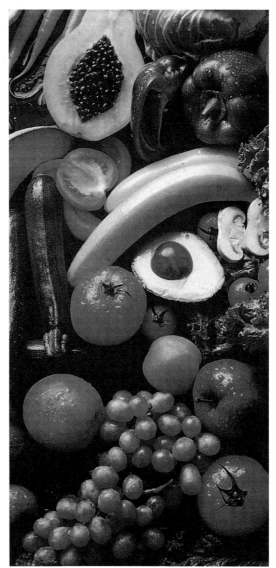

The medical profession has come a long way since the 1940s with the strong link between good nutrition and good health now universally acknowledged.

ahead of his time, too, in understanding the tremendous benefit of regular exercise, sunshine, daily bathing and fresh air to health.

Frankly, even now, too many of his profession underrate these factors and prefer to prescribe pills and super drugs rather than work at convincing patients of the wonders of natural cures and prevention which nature provides for free.

> *Even now, too many professionals prefer to prescribe pills and super drugs*

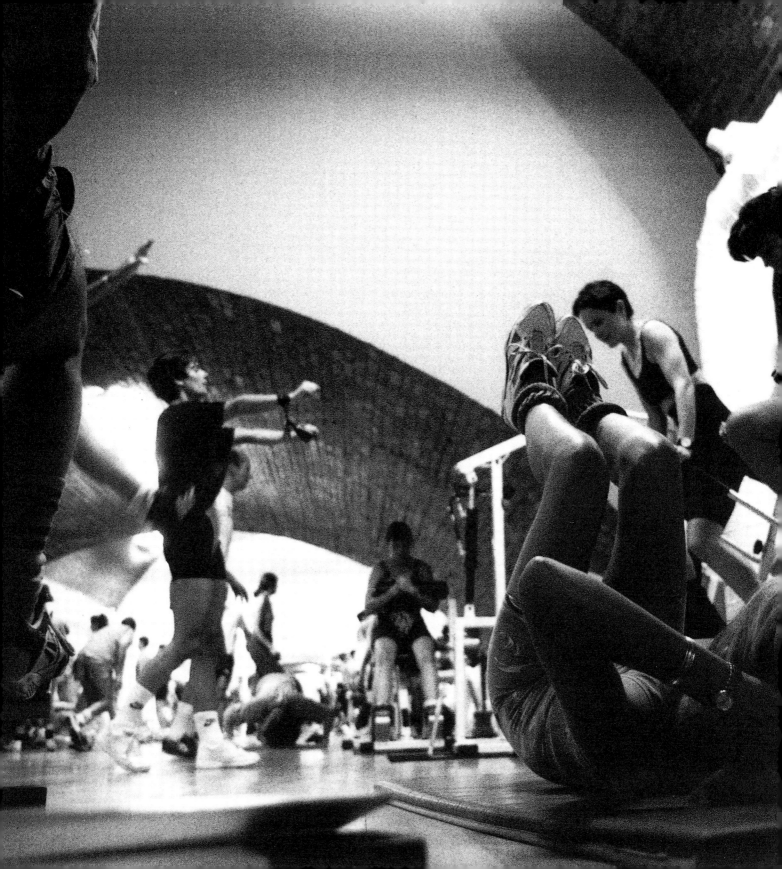

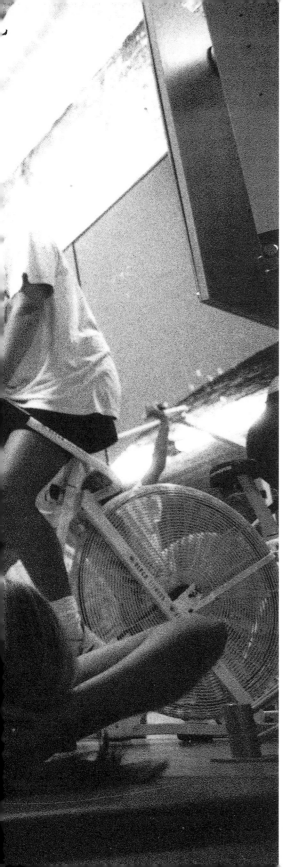

CHAPTER EIGHT

USE IT OR LOSE IT
THE VALUE OF REGULAR EXERCISE

'Use it or lose it' is an old adage that undoubtedly had its origins in the mythology which has evolved concerning the benefits of exercise.

Certainly, from earliest times, the value of regular physical training has been extolled and proven. On the other hand, it is beyond dispute that physical inactivity leads to a huge reduction in the efficiency of the body's functions and a decrease in its physical abilities.

There is so much evidence attesting to the positive and lasting effects of regular exercise, both physically and psychologically, that it would be a waste of time and effort to go to the trouble to prove the point again here.

Rather, I would prefer to assume our earlier chapters have so convinced you of the merits of a

> *There is so much evidence attesting to the lasting effects of regular exercise...*

healthy lifestyle that we can now concentrate upon the elements of a well-balanced training programme.

The basic elements of training

Actually there are four separate physical powers which need to be incorporated into your workouts if you are to develop a complete plan. These are:

1 Aerobic
(the single most important type for the non-athlete)
2 Resistance exercise
(trimming, toning, strengthening)
3 Stretching and relaxing
(yoga-type routines for increased flexibility)
4 Improving your anaerobic threshold
(how long you can sustain effort).

The first two are absolute necessities, the other two can be considered as optional.

As was pointed out earlier the genes we inherit not only dictate the shape of our bodies (which, in turn restricts the type of activities that are suitable), but I am afraid these inherited physical characteristics also limit the natural speed and/or stamina we are able to develop. Linford Christie and Carl Lewis, given their particular inherent physical dimensions and aptitudes, would never have been able to become world-class or even moderate performers over a mile, or a six-mile distance, nor could Seb Coe or Steve Ovett, with theirs, ever have excelled as sprinters.

When planning your own training programme you should take your own particular physical characteristics into account.

How basically to do it

Aerobic workouts

Aerobic training is easy, although some can find it boring. I do not, and I find it hard to understand others who do, as the challenge of the exercise is enthralling

to me. The sustaining of movement over a long period when your body wants to take the easy way out and just sit or lie down, is forever a contest between your mind and body. The satisfaction in being able to summon sufficient self control to delay the body's point of surrender provides a great, warm feeling, but I must add that this glow is not nearly as intense if the victory of will over want comes about by distraction (listening to a Walkman or watching television). This is not so much a win as a forfeit.

In fact the recent trend in some gymnasiums for installing televisions so that their members could be distracted by viewing television when doing their aerobic stints on the steps, cycles or treadmills, is to be lamented. If you are not concentrating, the body automatically slows and so such diversions are unsatisfactory on both counts – it is a terrible way to watch television and the aerobic workout is nowhere near as effective.

Training aerobically is really about non-stop movement. In aerobic classes you can combine this with resistance exercise, so for those short on time these classes are an ideal form of regular training. If you cannot attend them, or do not like them, then you have a choice between swimming, skipping, walking, jogging or running, cycling, stair-climbing or stepping. The aim is to take your heart rate level up to around the 130–150 beats per minute and maintain it there for anything from twenty minutes to one hour. The longer, the better.

It is the very length of the effort, not its difficulty, which many people find hard to maintain. Frankly it is a matter of determination, concentration and self-control. You will soon get used to it but, in the early stages, try to persevere for as long as you can, then drop the tempo if you must, before resuming. Never give in and stop completely – your body will have won and will continue to do so until your mind becomes strong enough to command and control. With the easy access I have to the facilities at Cannons, I find it

> *The sustaining of movement over a long period when your body wants to take the easy way out and just sit or lie down, is forever a contest between your mind and body*

helpful sometimes to do a bit of cross training. I work out first on the treadmill (starting with a brisk 15- to 20-minute walk up a five per cent incline, moving on to a 30- to 40-minute steady run gradually increasing in speed and tempo); next is 15 minutes on the step machine, a cycle and finally a swim. I can train non-stop for between 45 minutes and two hours in this way, pausing only to change activities. It is a great way to exercise aerobically and all these types of equipment are available at most gymnasiums.

Resistance exercise sessions

Two to three times a week you should add a resistance workout session. The point about this kind of workout is that your body needs at least a 48-hour rest before repeating the effort. Each set should be performed to the point of exhaustion (a state you should never reach during daily aerobic exercise) for that particular group of muscles' recommended sessions.

Later in the chapter we outline some examples of actual experiences and a regular workout you could well adopt, especially if you are just starting. We also make you aware of the differing benefits of the various types of aerobic activities.

We leave it to you to choose those which best suit your particular build and circumstances.

In my opinion too many books and references go to great lengths photographing and describing a vast number of exercises which, when examined closely, are all only slight variations from one another. Frankly these are mostly padding and we prefer in this publication to concentrate on giving you the pure basics. If you can do these consistently then that will be all you need to worry about. If possible repeat them, the same exercises, for years until they become routine.

Why should you need to vary them? They are easy to remember and the challenge is to improve the number you do week by week, or the weight you are able to heave until you reach a plateau at about 85

years of age. Then if you like you can begin to gradually reduce the intensity of repetitions and the actual poundage (or degree of resistance) in the weights. But only then. Routine is not necessarily boring and in fact, in my experience, soon after you start varying the types of movements being undertaken in your sessions, you often begin to miss the sessions themselves.

So, our recommendations are to always do some type of aerobic exercise each day for a minimum of 20 minutes – 45 minutes if you possibly can, and ideally an hour or so.

And then, additionally, three times a week you should be adding an exercise routine for your toning and strengthening.

These two types of workouts are complementary to each other and are both essential to any balanced health and fitness programme.

The optional additions to your weekly programme

The third and fourth elements to which we referred are not essential but do assist in the gaining of total fitness. So, for those of you who can fit in these types of sessions as well, we will also be showing how to undertake a type of yoga *stretching routine*. You would do these exercises on the alternate days to your resistance work. Again we have detailed only a set of basic movements which will be all you need to know in the first instance.

Finally, and especially if you are still active in sports competition of some kind, one or two of your aerobic sessions could be devoted into developing your anaerobic thresholds. Consequently we've also made some recommendations about how to go about this.

Be warned...

One note of caution here. Coaches often recommend workouts purportedly designed to improve anaerobic thresholds but which, although apparently easy, are

> *Do some type of aerobic exercise each day for a minimum of 20 minutes – 45 minutes if you possibly can, and ideally an hour or so*

quite dangerous. They seem easy because even though maximum effort is involved these efforts are interspersed with recovery periods.

Frankly, even in my best years when I was improving my personal best significantly, right through all distances from the 800 to the marathon, I rarely did this type of workout. When I did, it was limited to just once weekly.

Contrary to the beliefs of a number of coaches, I can testify that comparatively easy long aerobic training does strengthen your capacity to race at speed, as well as heightening aerobic thresholds, by improving the body's ability to circulate oxygen. I, and a number of my compatriots, proved it.

So, although later in this chapter we have described some interval and repetition type workouts for you, I repeat my caution against indulging too freely in them.

Working out in water

Towards the end of the section we have detailed some 'water workouts' which can replace your physical resistance routines if you have access to a suitable pool. For example, the water workouts can be very useful when travelling, as many hotels provide heated pools for guests, but very poor, if any, gymnasium equipment.

The advantages with water is that it is both multi-directional and supportive. It assists in resisting movement in any direction, whilst being protective of any jarring or sudden jerks.

Example of monthly record: Aerobic and Resistance Workouts.

20 Minute Circuit. Each circuit comprises 10 exercises, each to be repeated 10 times. Stop after 20 minutes and record the exact number of circuits and partial circuits that you have completed – e.g. if you complete 5 full circuits and 3 exercises of your final circuit, record 5.3

For your aerobic workouts simply record the type of activity with its initial and the duration – e.g. if you walked for 90 minutes, record W90; if you ran for 20 minutes, then R20; C for cycling, A for aerobics, S for swimming, SK for skipping, etc.

The record provides an easy reference to your progress and can be incorporated into a diary. You will be surprised how quickly improvement is made if training is consistent.

Month	Week 1		Week 2		Week 3		Week 3		Week 4		Week 5	
	CRCT	AER	CRCT	AER	CRCT	AER	CRCT	AER	CRCT	AER	CRCT	AER
Monday												
Tuesday												
Wednesday												
Thursday												
Friday												
Saturday												
Sunday												

Our actual excercise plan

The exercise plan we have detailed below consists of three structured workouts a week for six weeks to commence. If you already take exercise you should begin at the hardest level (week six) and continue from there, gradually increasing the number of repetitions and/or weights as you progress.

But for the beginners you should, as the start-up programme proceeds, increase the intensity and duration of the workouts.

Each exercise shown is itself simple to perform and requires little in the way of equipment. It is always best to read the instructions carefully before you begin so as to get to know the movements involved in the exercise thus avoiding an unnecessary waste of time or even injury. They have been designed to be implemented anywhere – in your living room or garage, office or hotel room. Wherever you are there should be no excuse for missing a session when it is due.

Instructions

refer to pp. 108 – 109 for diagrams and descriptions

1 The plan consists of resistance exercises performed with either a set of dumbbells, (five to ten pounds), a couple of house bricks, a Dynaband or, if you prefer, your own body weight. If you opt to use dumbbells purchase a set which can have additional weights added as you progress.

2 During the first two weeks, you should perform eight resistance exercises three times weekly and ten minutes of cardio-vascular daily. After two weeks, two more resistance exercises can be added and the duration of your daily cardio-vascular work should increase by five minutes, and again after a further two weeks so that in weeks five and six your workout consists of the ten resistance exercises for at least 20 minutes daily.

3 Each resistance exercise is to be performed for just ten repetitions, moving on to the next movement instantly.

4 When you are able to easily manage the required work rates, the resistance/intensity levels can be increased for the next workout. This can be done the following ways:

♥ Shortening the amount of rubber band being used.

♥ Increasing the weight of the dumbbells by adding extra 'plates'.

5 As soon as you have finished one exercise move quickly on to the next and so on through to the end of the workout.

6 The cardio-vascular section (aerobic sessions) of your training should always come after the resistance work.

Principles and practices

It is vital to realize that the two essential elements in a safe and effective weight programme are the regularity of the exercise regime itself, and the correct performance each movement to 'temporary muscular failure' (until you can truly do no more). Here are some rules:

1 Keep all movements *controlled*.

2 Work through a *full range of movement* in all exercises.

3 Do it right – strive to maintain correct technique at all times.

4 Allow 48 hours' rest between similar workouts.

5 Record your progress.

6 The session should never be more than 20 minutes.

7 Be intense – do not rest between exercises. 'Work hard, not long'.

9 Be regular, train three times a week on resistance work – no more, no less.

Aerobic or cardio-vascular training

It is important that your heart and lungs are exercised regularly. Activities such as cycling, stair-climbing, brisk walking, swimming, aerobic classes and running are ideal (choose activities you enjoy as this will help to

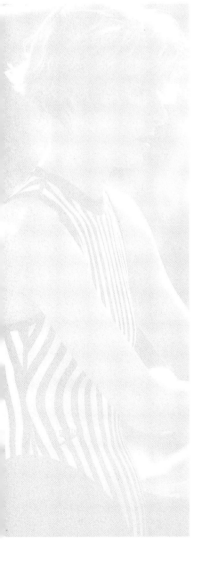

*10 repetitions of
each exercise in each
circuit. How many
circuits or part thereof
can you complete in 20
minutes? Limit to
three sessions weekly*
(at least 48 hours recovery
between sessions).

20 MINUTE CIRCUIT

1 *Twist Jumps (A)* Standing upright, jump up and twist in the air so that your feet land next to each other facing to the left with your upper torso facing to the right. Then jump again reversing your upper and lower body.

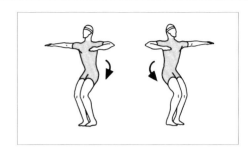

2 *Push Ups (C)* Full – Keep your hips and knees straight. Bend your elbows until your chest is approx 10cm from the floor.
Half – Bend your knees and lift your feet off the floor as shown. If you can, keep your thighs and upper body in a straight line.

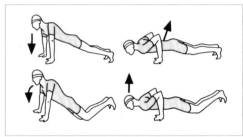

3 *Jumping Jacks (A)* From a standing start, jump up and simultaneously raise you hands above your head and spread your legs just beyond shoulder width to land. Keep your knees slightly bent to cushion the landing. The jump up again and return to start position.

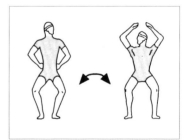

4 *Dips (C)* Place your hands near the edge of a step or chair with fingers pointing forwards. Bend your knees with your feet flat on the floor. Slowly bend your elbow to 90 degrees lowering your hips towards the floor and then return to straight arms.

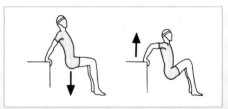

5 *High Knee Run (A)* Run on the spot, lift knee up to hip level with each stride. Count one each time your right knee reaches hip level.

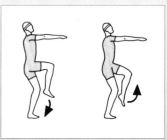

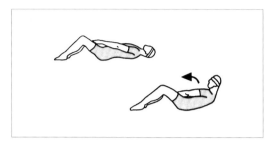

6 *Crunches (C)*

Lie with your back flat on the floor, knees bent, feet flat on the floor. Place your hands on your thighs. Slowly lift your head and shoulders, curling your upper torso forwards towards your knees. Keep your lower back in contact with the floor at all times.

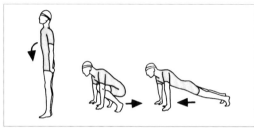

7 *Burpees (A)*

From a standing start, bend your knees and place your hands on the floor in front of you. Then in one movement throw your feet backwards and land with your legs straight out behind you. Immediately bring your feet back up towards your chest and stand upright.

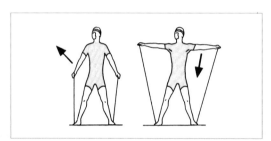

8 *Lateral Raise (C)*

Take a firm grip of each end of the Dynaband. Place your feet on the centre of the band and anchor to the floor. Keeping your body upright, raise your arms out to your sides until they reach shoulder level. Return your arms slowly to your sides.

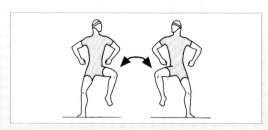

9 *Lateral Jumps (A)*

From a standing start, jump to the left and land on your left foot. Immediately jump to the right and land on your right foot. The motion is similar to a slalom skier. Count one each time you land on your right foot.

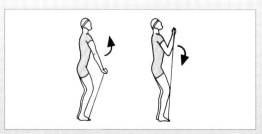

10 *Bicep Curl (C)*

Stand up, place one foot on the centre of the Dynaband anchoring it to the floor. Grasp an end in each hand, hold your arms straight down, with your hands resting on your upper thighs. Bend your arms at the elbow, slowly raise your hands towards your chest and return. Keep your body still throughout.

keep you motivated). The chart below shows just how beneficial each of these activities are.

The benefits of cardio-vascular training are:

♥ Lower heart rate – your resting and sub-maximal heart rate will decrease as less strain is placed on the heart during exercise.

♥ Lower blood pressure – this is extremely desirable as high blood pressure/hypertension is a major risk factor for heart disease.

♥ Oxygen extraction by the muscles from the circulating blood will improve, making your circulatory system more efficient.

♥ Stamina, or the ability to maintain work rate, will improve. It will become easier to maintain a high calorie-burning capability for longer, thus helping weight control.

♥ 'Burning' additional calories.

Note that the faster or more intense the effort, the greater the k/calories expended. Even so we recommend you do not extend yourself during any cardio-vascular activity so much that you become breathless (as distinct from breathing heavily but under control). Normally this means keeping your heartbeats per minute to 160 or less. Aim for gradual improvement and measure by time and mileage where relevant.

K/calories expended for five, ten, twenty and thirty minutes of activity

You should be aiming to expend around 200–600 k/calories per session, six to seven times a week to gain the proper benefit from this type of exercise. As you can see when examining the chart, running is by far the quickest, and I feel the easiest, way of achieving this.

	5 mins	10 mins	20 mins	30 mins
Walking (4mph/15 mins per mile)	25	50	100	150
Horseback riding (walk/gallop)	15/50	30/100	60/200	90/300
Cycling (13mph)	25/50	50/100	100/200	150/300
Dancing	25/40	50/80	100/160	150/300
Gymnastics (aerobics)	25/40	50/80	100/160	150/240
Tennis	35/50	70/100	140/200	210/300
Squash	50/60	100/120	200/240	300/360
Football	45	90	180	270
Rowing (sculling)	30	60	120	180
Gardening	25	50	100	150
Swimming breaststroke	30/60	60/120	120/240	180/360
backstroke	25/50	50/100	100/200	150/300
freestyle	25/50	50/100	100/200	150/300
Jogging (9 mins per mile)	50	100	200	300
Running (6 mins per mile)	100	200	400	600
Climbing	50/60	100/120	200/240	300/360
Skiing	50/100	100/200	200/240	300/360

The faster or more intense the effort, the greater the k/calories expended.

Stretching routine (see pp. 112 – 117)

We recommend this programme on the days of the week on which you do not do the resistance workout.

It is a relaxing series, based on the yoga movements, which stretch, tone and relax various muscle groups. There is no need to worry about the yoga breathing techniques which accompany these movements when they are incorporated into a yoga class. Just concentrate on breathing normally, inhaling on the easy or negative phase, and exhaling on the positive or effort-promoting phase.

Gradually increase repetitions until you are doing ten for each movement, all of them slowly and easily. You will be amazed at how quickly you improve your body tone if you can keep this routine going.

High intensive workouts

The best book I have seen on the subject of the effect of workouts is a 1989 publication originally from Finland called *Training Lactate Pulse Rate* by Dr Peter Janssen, a Dutch endurance athlete and sports medicine expert, who has specialized in the research of

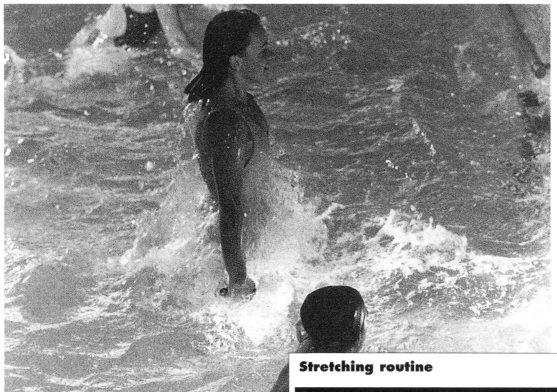

> *Aim for gradual improvement and measure by time and mileage where relevant*

Stretching routine

Exercise description	Muscle groups worked	Weeks 1&2	Weeks 3&4	Weeks 5&6
Body roll	Waist, neck and balance	4 4	6 6	8 8
Standing side bend	Buttocks, sides, thighs and back	4 4	6 6	8 8
Midriff toner	Lower back, abdomen and sides	4	6	8
Squat	Legs and thighs	4	6	8
The bow	Arms, shoulders, neck and chest	-	4	6
The coil	Spine, neck, buttocks and thighs	-	4	6
Front push-up	Shoulders, arms and waist	-	-	4
The plough	Back muscles	-	-	4

The body roll

Tones waist muscles and releases neck tension. Bend from waist, not the hips.

1 Stand with the legs and feet together and grip your waist with your hands.

2 Push the pelvis forward a little and bend over from the waist.

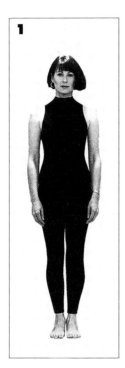
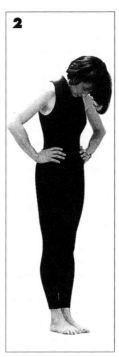
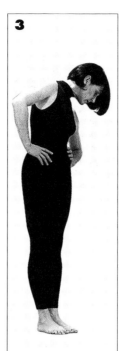
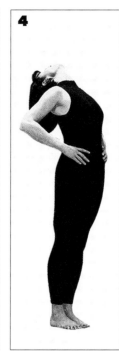

3 Slowly roll the top half of your body around to your left and hold it for a few seconds.

4 Continue on around to the back, allowing the head to go back a little and making sure that the shoulders are back and down. Hold for a few seconds.

5 Carry on rolling around to your right, and again hold the position for a few seconds.

6 Slowly return to the front, then repeat rotation once more to the left before relaxing like this.

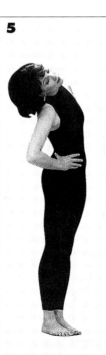
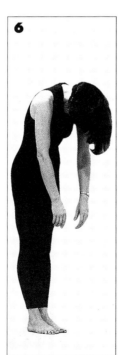
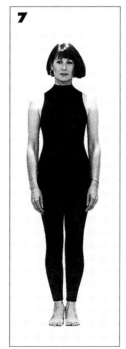

7 Straighten up slowly, ready to execute the movement twice round to the right.

Standing side bend

Stretches the sides of the body and waist area. Slide your hand down your leg as you bend.

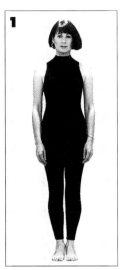 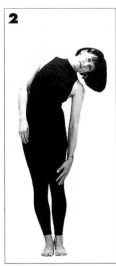 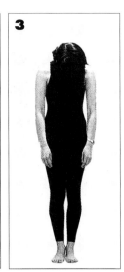 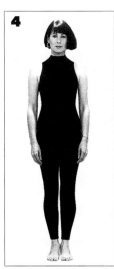

1 Stand straight with the legs and feet together and the head erect. Place the palms of the hands flat against the legs.

2 Slowly bend over to the right, sliding the right hand down towards the knee. Your left hand will automatically slide up towards the hip. Allow your head to relax right over. Hold in your comfortable position for five.

3 Straighten up slowly, pushing down with your left hand to help you. The head comes up only when the body is straight again.

4 Gently relax the head over for a few seconds before repeating on the other side. Then repeat entire movement again, once each side.

Midriff toner

Keeps spine supple and strong while toning waist muscles. Elbows should be straight throughout the movement.

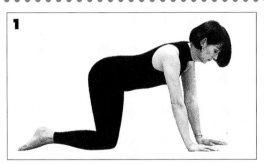

1 Kneel, arms rigid, back straight, thighs at right-angles to calves, toes pointing back.

2 Slowly let the back sink down, pushing bottom right up and out.

3 Raise the face and see as much of the ceiling as you can. Hold the position for a count of five.

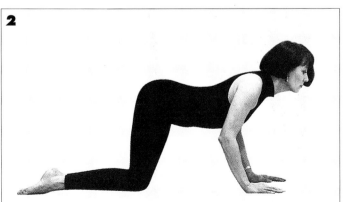

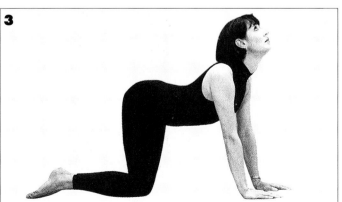

Midriff toner (cont.)

4 Now slowly reverse the position by arching the back and gently pushing the pelvis forward.

5 Try to get the chin right down on to the chest. Hold position for a count of five and immediately repeat entire movement.

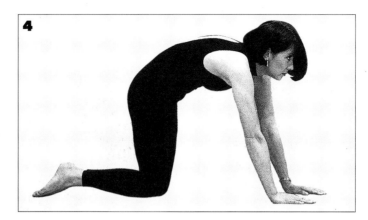

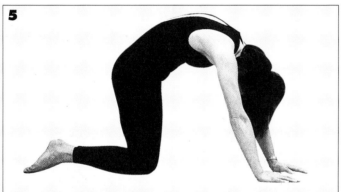

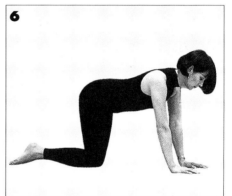

6 Return to original position and relax for a few moments, then repeat once more.

The Squat

Assists with balance and posture while strengthening knee and Achilles tendons. Ideal exercise for runners – hold your heels on the floor for as long as possible, keep knees together throughout the movement if you can.

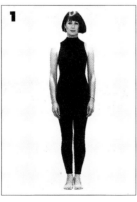

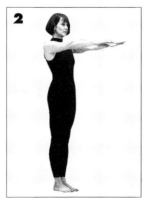

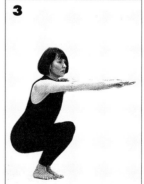

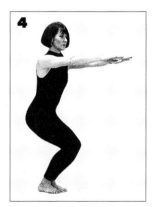

1 Stand with your back straight, your head erect and your legs and feet together.

2 Raise arms level with shoulders, turning palms of hands towards the floor.

3 Keeping back straight, slowly bend knees and come on to the balls of the feet.

4 Straighten up slowly, ready to repeat.

The Bow

This is not an easy movement, especially for men, but it is possible with patience and it does strengthen the back and chest muscles. If you cannot reach both feet, as in No.3, try taking one foot at a time until it is possible to get two.

1 Lie flat, arms along sides, face down with chin supporting head.

2 Start to bend the knees bringing the feet in towards the body.

3 When the feet are as close as they will go, reach back with the hands and try to take the feet.

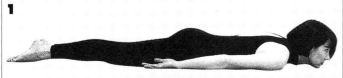

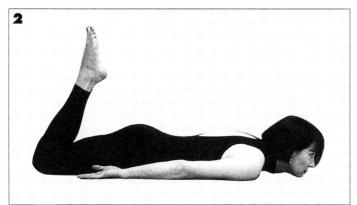

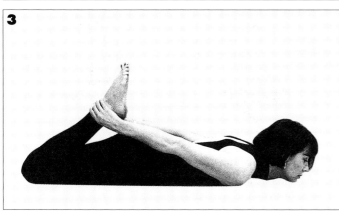

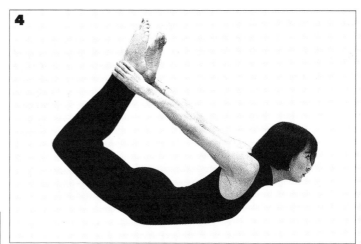

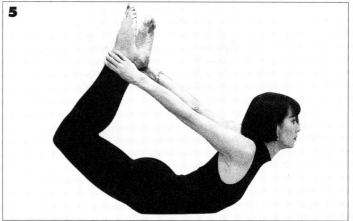

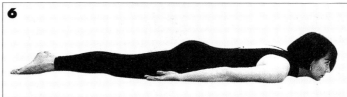

4 Keeping the elbows straight, start to raise the head.

5 Gently push feet towards floor pulling shoulders back – then look up to ceiling as much as you can. Hold position for a count of five.

6 Let your body sink down until your face is resting on the chin. Only release feet when they won't spring out of the hands too much. Lower your legs to the floor, relax at the beginning pose, wait a few seconds and repeat.

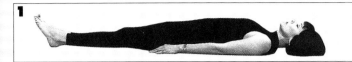

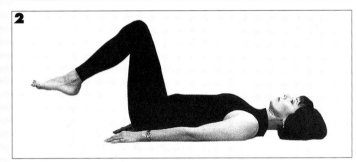

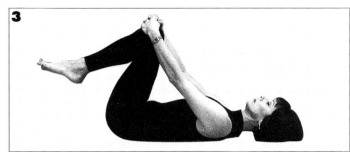

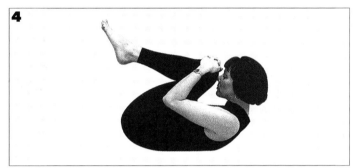

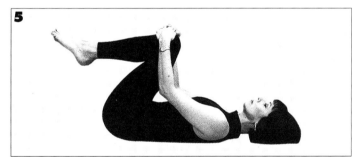

The Coil

Ensures strength and mobility in the neck while toning the buttocks and abdominals. Make certain elbows stay pointing towards the floor.

1 Lie with the legs and feet together and the palms of the hands towards the floor.

2 Raise legs, keeping the knees straight and the feet together.

3 Interlock the fingers and loop the hands over the knees.

4 Pull on the knees with the hands and raise your head towards the knees. Hold the position for a count of five.

5 Lower the head to the floor and relax like this for a few seconds before repeating.

Push-up

Strengthens the forearms, arms and shoulders. Useful for stretching of hamstrings and Achilles tendons.

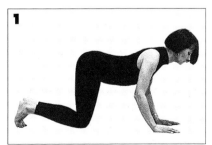

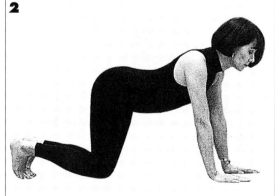

1 On hands and knees try to place hands directly below shoulders. Tuck toes under so that you are resting on balls of feet.

2 Push up, straightening elbows and-knees, and allow head to relax completely – hang. Hold position for a count of five.

The Plough

Stretches and strengthens back and abdominal muscles. Move slowly at all times.

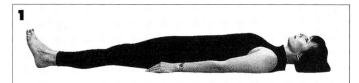

1 Bring the legs and feet together and turn the palms of the hands towards the floor.

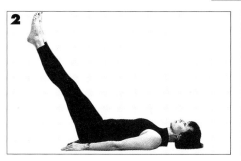

2 Raise your legs, keeping the knees straight and the feet together.

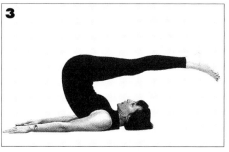

3 Bring the legs over as far as they will go comfortably. Hold the position for five.

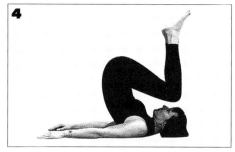

4 Come out of plough by bending knees in to chest and tucking feet in — in tight ball.

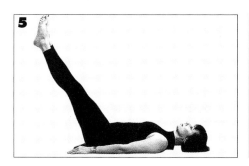

5 Slowly roll out, extending the legs on the way.

6 Bring the legs smoothly back down to the floor and relax in the 'corpse' position for a few seconds before repeating.

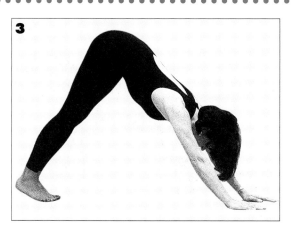

3 Slowly lower knees and return to your starting position. (Pressing the knees together as you lower will help you to come down slowly and smoothly.) The head can stay relaxed forward while you wait a few seconds before repeating.

4 After executing the movement twice, relax this position to allow the body to unwind.

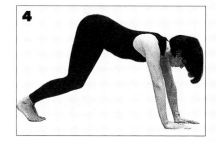

anaerobic thresholds and the effect of different lactate levels upon training and performance. As workload increases the working muscles produce more and more lactic acid. Too much acidity in the body prevents its proper operation but, in normal circumstances, the fit athlete disposes of this lactic acid by his/her oxygen replenishment systems.

But once a certain speed or effort is reached there is a crossover between the aerobic and anaerobic zones, when the oxygen being circulated can no longer cope with the unusual measures of lactic acid in the blood. This is expressed by the unit millimoles per litre (mM/l). Healthy people, at rest, have between 1mM/l and 2mM/l at all times. The usual level beyond which the body will not function is around 4mM/l and the crossover point between aerobic and anaerobic exertion can vary from 1.5 to 4mM/l.

The fitter you are, the more efficiently your aerobic system is operating, the higher this figure is before the crossover. Training aerobically can improve it by up to 100% (from 1.5mM/l to 3mM/l, for example).

The other way to combat nature is to build the body's resistance to high lactate value. Four-hundred-metre runners must try to do this as they would never be able to run their race fast enough to be competitive if they were to stay within normal aerobic capacity.

There is a method by which to artificially check this anaerobic threshold called the Conconi test, which claims 99% accuracy. It is a practical impossibility to take blood samples and check the lactate presence so the Conconi method has been developed as the most accurate simulated way of establishing this threshold.

The ability of an athlete to discover his or her lactate tolerance involves stress testing at full speed, usually on an indoor bicycle or treadmill which can measure output. The table on the left shows the average relative anaerobic thresholds of various types of athletes from sprinters to marathon runners. Natural sprinters enter oxygen debt and begin to accumulate lactose in their muscles at a much slower pace (at three metres per second compared to five metres per second of distance runners) and at a lower level (3.17mM/l to the 4.89mM/l of marathon runners). Yet they also develop an ability to operate more efficiently for longer whilst combating this oxygen debt.

Variation of anaerobic thresholds in different athletic types

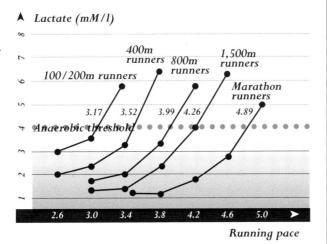

Running pace and anaerobic threshold in various top-class female athletes. The graph shows averages from different size groups of top-class German runners.

Variation of workloads before anaerobic threshold is reached

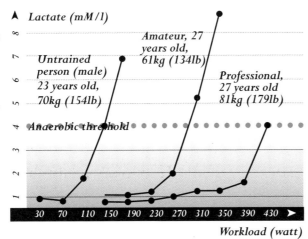

Differences in performance, assessed according to the height of the anaerobic threshold, with increasing workload in a bicycle ergometric exercise test.

The effect of high lactate levels

The first effect of high lactate levels is a feeling of tiredness in the muscles. This is followed by a drop off in skills, especially in sports such as tennis, squash or soccer. Training should not take place if players are recovering from a hard effort, be it a match or a physical workout which has left levels of 6mM/l or more. Their physical co-ordination would be so disturbed that the practising of skills would only lead to a deterioration of confidence and would have no positive effect.

High lactate values also increase the risk of injury, especially with micro ruptures, which often cause more serious injuries such as muscle tears or strains later. In addition, the system which propels sprinters, the creatine phosphate system, is disturbed by high lactate formation. This is a very good reason to avoid such occurrences during sprint training.

Lastly, oxidation stagnates – the glycogen stores would have been depleted to cause the retention of lactic acid in the body and, while this lactate value remains high, oxidation is slow and energy supply dwindles to nothing until the lactate value drops, with rest, and the glycogen stores begin to be replenished.

Training on pulse rates

Once the anaerobic threshold is established it is possible to determine the most effective pulse rate at which training can be conducted. This is because the pulse rate at which the threshold occurs can be considered to be the maximum rate for aerobic type workouts. There are two types of training which will:

a increase this anaerobic threshold and thus raise aerobic ability

b train the body to greater lactic acid tolerance.

The chart demonstrates this graphically.

For speed endurance

In training the body's tolerance to high lactate levels the best system would appear to be interval workouts with

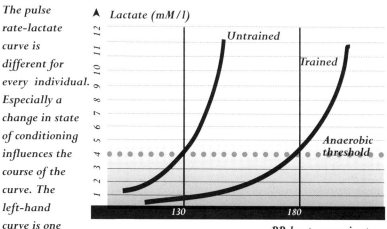

Variation of anaerobic thresholds in different athletic types

The pulse rate-lactate curve is different for every individual. Especially a change in state of conditioning influences the course of the curve. The left-hand curve is one of an untrained person.

Lactate (mM/l)

Untrained

Trained

Anaerobic threshold

130   180

PR beats per minute

His deflection point is at a PR of 130 beats per minute. The right-hand curve shows that after a period of training, the PR at the deflection point has shifted to 180 beats per minute.

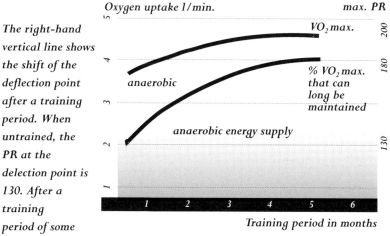

Variation of workloads before anaerobic threshold is reached

The right-hand vertical line shows the shift of the deflection point after a training period. When untrained, the PR at the delection point is 130. After a training period of some months the deflection point shifts to 180 beats per minute.

Oxygen uptake l/min.   max. PR

VO_2 max.

anaerobic

% VO_2 max. that can long be maintained

anaerobic energy supply

1   2   3   4   5   6

Training period in months

> *Aqua workouts are not a soft training option. Many Olympic athletes use an aqua programme to improve performance*

exertions from 20–180 seconds followed by recoveries of 30–60 seconds. It is interesting that Dr Janssen asserts that the recovery period should not be too long as the lactate content 'must not decrease too much' (this apparently destabilizes the system and encourages acidity in muscles). The good doctor, as I do, raises the danger signals on this type of workout. My experience with sessions such as 12 x 400 metres in say 55–56 seconds for each 400 has been disastrous. Mainly, I think it comes about from the tendency to repeat such sessions too soon or to run each positive effort too fast.

For power and acceleration

There is one other type of physical fitness training – that is, other than for athletic skills. It is for the creatine phosphate system – muscle speed. Dr Janssen's work isolates the best type of training for this as well. Namely he recommends that training *for speed* (the creatine phosphate system) should concentrate on five- to ten- or twenty-second maximal efforts with complete recoveries so that the lactate has always returned to below its crossover point between efforts. Once again this recovery can best be detected by checking that the pulse rate has come back to below 120 beats per minute (twenty beats in ten seconds).

My experience

My preference has always been to have a session of short sprints or surges with similar quick recoveries. In fact this type of workout was my only track session whilst I was competing between 1965 and 1970. It now seems, from Dr Janssen's evidence, we had chanced upon what was apparently the best type of training we could have chosen to complement the consistently long endurance running at about 70% MHR (maximum heart rate).

What proportion of the training should easy aerobic, speed endurance and power running form?

Unfortunately, Dr Janssen becomes a little too detailed in his book and provides endless tables and recommendations on what speed to run when and the proportion of time runners, cyclists and swimmers should devote to the three differing types of training.

I believe it is sufficient here to make you aware of the anaerobic threshold method and to recommend that you pay attention to it when devising your aerobic workouts. If you do not wish to be too scientific then revert back to our earlier recommen-dations – that is to do anything from 20–60 minutes daily of non-stop aerobic work. You cannot go too wrong with this.

If you walk in these workouts walk briskly, do not merely stroll. If you jog or run take care. You should never be breathless – just run easily and don't be ashamed to walk occasionally if you feel distressed at any time. Cycling falls somewhere between the comfort of walking and the difficulty of running. You should do it at around 80% effort. Swimming is a matter of style – if you are a good swimmer then lap steadily. If you are not so good then take care to intersperse freestyle with breaststroke whenever you are feeling that you are over exerting. Stop and take your pulse frequently (taking ten-second counts) to be certain you are not overtaxing yourself. If you count more than 25 beats in those ten-second pauses then you should ease down a little. Probably your count will be somewhere between 20 and 25, that is, 120–170 beats per minute.

There is no doubt, of all the differing types of exercise, those based on aerobic endurance are the most beneficial for your physiology and especially for the health of your heart. And there are so many ways of combining these that only your own imagination, and any limitation of facilities, should restrict you.

We are assuming you are intelligent enough to select those workouts which best suit your physique and temperament, and, if still active, your particular sport. I do stress though, it is most important that a foundation of aerobic fitness, easy long running and/or cycling, is the surest path to fitness of any sort. Despite the proof, most coaches and phys. eds. recommend a preponderance of interval and repetition work. They are wrong.

Pools are useful for other exercise besides just swimming

Aqua fitness

Aqua aerobics, is not just an old ladies' class performed to slow relaxing music. Indeed, it is a fact that water has been used as a medium of exercise throughout history beginning in the years Before Christ with the Greeks and Romans. The Chinese, too, have always been aware of the merits of water resistance for strengthening and recuperation. Nowadays aqua exercise is fast becoming one of the most enjoyable fitness trends of the 1990s as its versatility allows participants of varying abilities to achieve an effective workout. Water exercise offers a challenging option for individuals interested in general fitness, injury rehabilitation, and low impact or cross training.

How does it work and why?

Once in water the body becomes almost weightless and movements that are impossible on land become possible. Resistance is the key to water fitness. Water provides twelve times more resistance to work against than air. What is more, this resistance is multi-directional rather than uni-directional, and allows the working of opposing muscle groups during the same exercise. When in the water, movements performed create drag and turbulence. If you speed these up, then the resistance increases, making your muscles work harder. However, *unlike working out normally, slow movements are not effective,* as you will just be working with the buoyancy of the water.

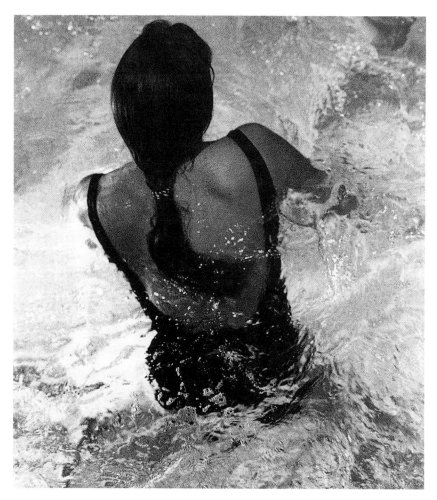

Benefits

One of the major benefits is that approximately 80% of impact stress on the joints and bones is absorbed by the water. Water workouts also promote a more efficient blood circulation, as the water pressure helps the blood to flow more easily. And a more efficient circulation means that more oxygen is absorbed which reduces the heart's workload.

Depending on the specific goals of the routine, water workouts provide excellent cardio-vascular training with added toning and strength benefits. Abdominal and back muscles are constantly contracting so

Aquatic exercise is fast becoming one of the most important workout options due to its versatility and effectiveness.

Continually push and pull the water to create maximum resistance

there is no need to concentrate on specific abdominal exercises.

Moreover, because of the water's buoyancy, exercise programmes are more appealing to less co-ordinated people. Water aids circulation and its massaging effects help to reduce cellulite.

Different types of exercising in the water

Over the last few years a number of types of equipment and different clothing have been developed specifically to create even more resistance in the water. Varying from dumbbells to webbed gloves, these added extras will really get you into shape.

Water workout exercises 1 ARMS

Start your workout with the knees bent, feet shoulder-width apart and shoulders just below the water line.

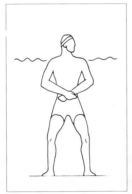

Criss-Cross Arms – *alternately, cross arms at wrists.*

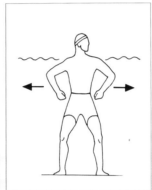

Triceps Extension – *with elbows bent and raised, extend arms out to the sides and back.*

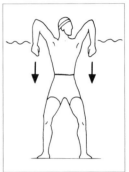

Upright Row – *with elbows bent and lifted high towards the surface, push fists down through water.*

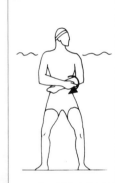

Rolling – *roll forearms around one another, first forwards then backwards.*

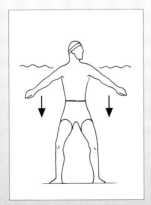

Lateral Press – *extend arms fully to sides, push down with open hands, crossing arms in front of the body before raising them.*

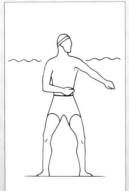

Alternate Arm Punches – *forward, to the sides and down through the water.*

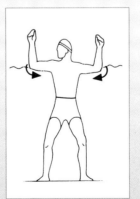

Chest & Back Press – *with elbows bent 90 degrees at shoulder height, alternately press elbows together then back.*

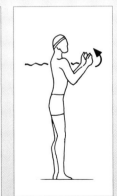

Biceps Curl – *with elbows bent, open and close hands as you pull up and push down through the water.*

Most people view aqua aerobic exercises as exclusively for women but at Cannons our experience, particularly with classes such as aqua circuits, is that they are attended by as many men as women.

Aqua step is another type of workout that has recently appeared in some pools although many 'land steppers' feel that aqua step is not as beneficial or intense as land-based steps. It has its own charm and intensities and certainly does not cause the same number of joint problems or muscle stiffness.

Another type of popular water workout is deep water exercise. Using a buoyancy belt and optional

Water workout exercises 2 LOWER BODY

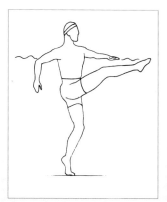

High Kicks — with knees bent, alternately high kick through the water using arms for balance.

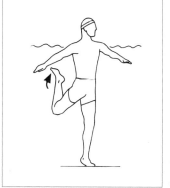

Hamstring Curl — with weight on left leg, arms outstretched, repeatedly lift right heel to buttock. Change leg.

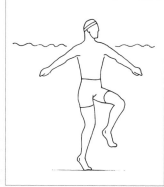

Skateboarding — weight on left leg, arms outstretched, repeatedly skateboard in the water. Change leg.

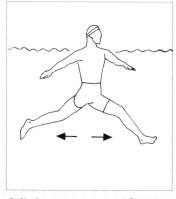

Split Jump — starting and finishing with both feet together, jump into forward splits.

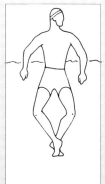

Cross Leg Jump — feet shoulder-width apart, jump high out of the water, crossing legs before landing

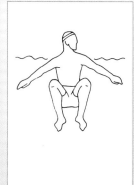

Tuck Jump — jump with both feet off the ground and knees tucked up towards chest. Use arms to maintain balance.

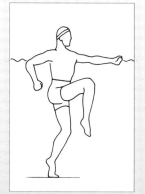

High Knee Jog — fast as possible, jog on the spot, knees lifted high towards the surface alternately punching the water with clenched fists.

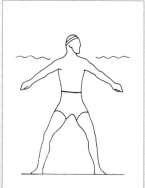

Star Jump (Low) — jump with both feet off ground, knees tucked up towards chest, land with feet wide apart. Repeat.

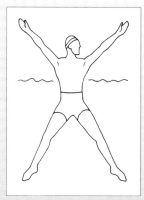

Star Jump (High) — jump high out of the water with arms and legs wide apart, returning to normal starting position on landing.

ankle cuffs a whole workout can be achieved in the deep end of the pool. Deep water aqua is great for improving posture, muscle tone and flexibility, as the water gently stretches tendons and muscles.

How to get the most benefit from your workout

The illustrations, here and on the previous pages, show some recommended routines for you to try.

Getting used to moving in water takes time. You should practise moving to and fro and using your arms to pull you before attempting any routines. When performing power moves ensure that your shoulders are under water and you are in a squat or lunge position. This will make you more stable and allow you to perform dynamic moves more effectively.

When jogging in water push your heels down, as running on your toes may lead to cramp and sore calf muscles. Do not move softly in the water, take hold of it and thrust. Continually push and pull the water to create maximum resistance. When jumping, land with bent knees to disperse impact through the joints.

Aqua workouts are not a soft training option. Many Olympic athletes use an aqua programme in training to improve performance. World martial arts champion, Geoff Thompson, and tennis star, Martina Navratilova, have long trained in the water to develop flexibility, speed and strength without risk of injury.

Water°workout exercises   3 ABDOMINALS AND TORSO

Twists – with a slight spring from both feet, twist torso to left and right as quickly as possible keeping arms close to your sides. Repeat more slowly with arms stretched out wide.

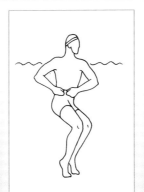

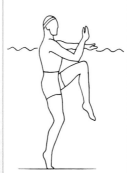

Alternate Elbows to Knees – alternately touch left elbow to right knee and right elbow to left knee using free arm to maintain balance.

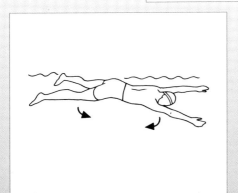

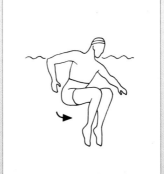

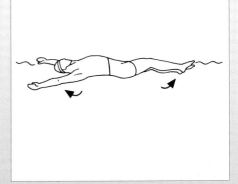

Reverse Stretch – from a fully stretched floating position facing the water, draw outstretched arms down and back and knees towards the chest into a tuck position. Push feet forwards and arms back above the head finishing in a fully stretched floating position facing the ceiling.

Water workout exercises   4 GENERAL

Breast Stroke Arms *– elbows bent and arms together in front of chest, push open hands forwards until fully extended, sweep arms wide and out to sides. Draw them back into the starting position.*

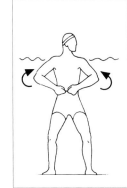

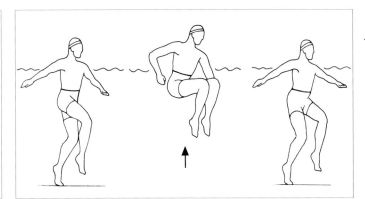

Lunge Jump *– from lunge position and with arms out- stretched, spring off leading foot, drawing knees towards chest into tuck position. Change leading leg before landing again in the lunge.*

Frog Jump *– both knees slightly bent, shoulder-width apart, repeatedly spring high out of water, lifting heels up and out to sides. Pull down outstretched arms to aid propul- sion. Land in normal starting position.*

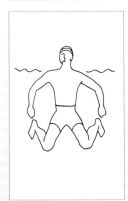

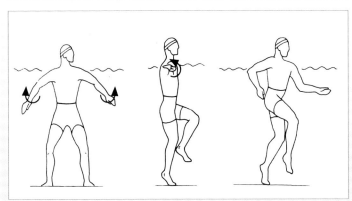

Wrist Circling *– with elbows slightly bent and outstretched palms, repeatedly sweep hands in small circles in the water by rotating first the left and then the right wrist.*

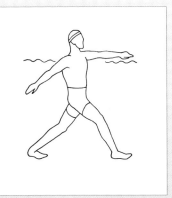

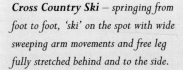

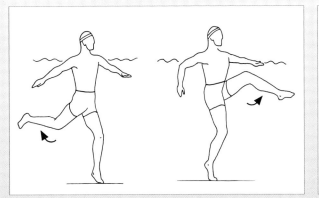

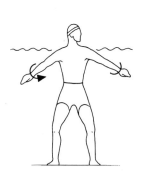

Cross Country Ski *– springing from foot to foot, 'ski' on the spot with wide sweeping arm movements and free leg fully stretched behind and to the side.*

Rocking Horse *– with both knees slightly bent and one leg in front of the other, rock back and forth with a slight spring off the bottom of the pool and arms outstretched for balance. Change lead- ing leg and repeat.*

Arm Circling *– with arms fully extend- ed to the sides and palms facing down, repeatedly draw circles in the water, first forwards then backwards.*

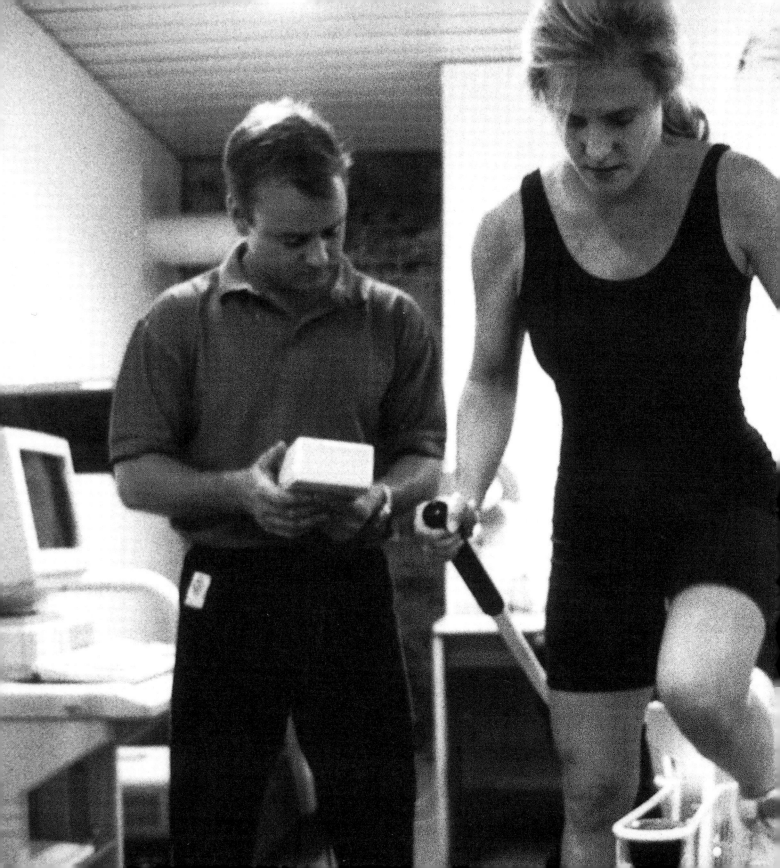

CHAPTER NINE

KEEPING TRACK MONITORING PROGRESS

It has always been a constant source of amazement to me why so many people choose not to know how healthy or fit they are as long as 'everything is working all right'.

The same people would not dream of waiting for their car to break down before having it serviced, or running a business without periodic and regular reports on its health and progress.

I think the medical profession itself is partly to blame by making health screens and other periodic medical check-ups so complex and expensive on the one hand, and mundane and ineffective on the other.

For example most large firms expect their chief executives to pass yearly medical examinations but, until recent years, these were so routine that if the personnel concerned could still breathe and walk 100 metres in two minutes, they were given the all clear.

This is like the car mechanic listening to the

> *People would not dream of waiting for their car to break down before having it serviced*

engine, checking the oil and petrol, and saying your vehicle should be good for another 10,000 miles.

Consequently we feel it is important that you not only check your state of health annually, but take care to select and regularly undertake the type of fitness tests and health screens which fit your particular lifestyle. Make certain these are both pertinent and effective. Here are some which you should consider:

The fundamental four

As a matter of routine everyone should get to know how they stand in relation to what we call the fundamental four measurements:

♥ Blood cholesterol, including HDL ratio
  (HDL = high density lipoproteins)
♥ Blood pressure
♥ Body fat percentage
♥ Oxygen uptake index.

In our opinion these are all dynamic measurements. The need to check blood pressure is obvious and the importance of both cholesterol and the proportion of HDL to LDL (low density lipoproteins) discussed by Dr Briffa on page 26.

I do not think anybody would query the inclusion of these in our fundamental four but they may ask why you need to know how fat people are or how efficient is their cardio-respiratory system.

These are included because they are both early warning measurements. You may not have high blood pressure yet and your cholesterol count could be okay too, but if you are overweight and inefficient in circulating oxygen, then you can be pretty sure you are heading for trouble soon. They are the equivalent of having early warning indicators in a civil defence system. It is all very well to ensure everything is working well back home in the last line of defence, but it is equally important to develop long-range lookouts — ways to detect enemy intrusion at its sources. This is exactly the role these two tests perform. Both are

volatile and subject to relatively quick improvements if the subject decides not to risk further deterioration, and to do something to arrest or improve his or her condition.

We suggest these tests are undertaken quarterly or, if you are young and fit, half yearly. Not longer.

Anaerobic threshold

This dynamic test is discussed in the previous chapter on exercise (see p. 118). Only relatively recently has it been possible to calculate this important measurement for those who are serious about their training.

It provides both a guide to the level at which training can be maximized and an indication how best to use your own pulse rates for this purpose.

Power and speed endurance tests

Also important for active athletes, especially those involved in speed sports such as squash, tennis, soccer, rugby, badminton, etc. They provide a good indication of both progress and potential.

Well-man and well-woman screens

At the other end of the scale are the general health screens everyone should have annually after 40.

These should include:

♥ Medical/lifestyle history
♥ Physical examination
♥ Complete pathology analysis consisting of: haematology, urinalysis and biochemistry (cholesterol, liver and kidney function)
♥ Body composition analysis utilizing skinfold measurements
♥ Exercise tolerance test (maximal/submaximal) on motorized treadmill or cycle ergometer with multi-lead ECG and blood pressure monitoring
♥ Back care functional evaluation, testing strength and flexibility in muscle groups which can influence the incidence of back pain

If you're overweight and inefficient in circulating oxygen, you can be pretty sure you're heading for trouble soon

♥ Lung function test to screen for possible respiratory disorders

♥ Resting ECG

♥ Gross vision test

♥ Hearing test

♥ Exercise prescription

♥ Discussion of evaluation results and recommendations with doctor and exercise physiologist

♥ Comprehensive report on evaluation results and recommendations

♥ Counselling information kit

♥ Early detection cancer X-rays and examinations.

Specific tests

Then there another number of specific tests that can be taken individually, such as:

♥ Blood pressure

♥ Heart ECG at risk and sub-maximum exertion levels

♥ Various muscle groups, especially the lower back

♥ Complete pathology analysis incorporating blood, urine and biochemistry to check cholesterol, liver and kidney functions

♥ Vision

♥ Hearing

♥ Anaerobic threshold

♥ VO2 maximum (aerobic function)

♥ X-ray and cancer scans.

Reports

Each test should result in a comprehensive report and be explained in full by the organization and practitioners responsible. Any questions should be answered in full and most will include recommendations on overcoming any weaknesses that have been detected.

Employers' responsibilities

How much better it would be if governments and employers were able to get behind these sort of dynamic tests and health screens with a plan to have the population tested or screened in this way. Prevention is always less expensive than treatment but, for some reason, such a concept is still anathema to the bureaucrats who control public spendin, and employers, in the main, look at the costs of such programmes (which can be easily spotted in the account books) rather than reviewing the benefits. These are usually higher than the costs, but much harder to evaluate or detect as they are reflected in employees' attitudes, productivity and regularity of attendance.

"Prevention is always less expensive than treatment but such a concept is still anathema to the bureaucrats who control public spending and policy"

LIFESTYLE QUESTIONNAIRE

In order to assess your current state of health and fitness we have provided, on the following pages, a series of self-assessments and tests.

The results should be tabled on the chart at the end of the questionnaire. Each of the assessments set out on the following pages has a rating and a score which can be recorded on the chart provided.

We have given you enough space to complete three tests – and these should be done perhaps three to six months apart, so that you can trace your progress in any of the programmes you undertake.

We have not attempted to try to establish any sort of overall rating but rather a system to allow you to rate yourself in each aspect of your lifestyle and scale of fitness – using the letters 'A' to 'G' with 'A' being outstanding, then down the scale to 'G' which indicates urgent action is needed.

On the pages following the tests are the score sheets. For some of the tests it will help if you have the assistance of a partner.

1 We start with the resting heart rate

This deteriorates with age. Take your pulse, either at the wrist or neck using your fingertips (never the thumb) for a minute after waking in the morning and then score yourself as in the chart overleaf:

Rating Resting heart rate	Age Range					
	18–25	*26–35*	*36–45*	*46–55*	*56–65*	*66–99*
A Oustanding	55	54	56	57	56	55
B Superior	61	61	62	63	61	61
C Above average	65	65	66	67	67	65
D Average	69	70	70	71	71	69
E Below average	73	74	76	76	75	73
F Fair	81	81	82	83	81	79
G Poor	120	120	120	120	120	120

1 RESULT (Heart beats per minute)

RATING ....

2 Your medical history

Have you, your parents, siblings or children had an of
the following diagnosed by a doctor?
If yes please indicate with a tick.

Medical history	Myself	Relative
Heart disease or attack		
High blood pressure		
Stroke		
Cancer (please specify)		
Diabetes		
High cholesterol		

2 RESULT (Number of ticks)

RATING ....

Rating Medical history	Number of ticks
A Outstanding	0
B Above average	2+
C Average	4+
D Below average	6+
E Poor	8+
F Close attention needed	10+

Thirdly let's look at your bad habits:

Alcohol and Tobacco use

How many units of alcohol/cigarettes do you
drink/smoke usually in a week/day:

3 Tobacco

Rating	Number of cigarettes/day
A No problem	0
C Minimal risk	1
D Moderate risk	5
F Dangerous	10
G Deadly	20

3 RESULT (Number of cigarettes per day)

RATING ....

4 Alcohol

How many units of alcohol do you drink in a week:

Bottles or half pints of beer per week ....

Glasses of wine or champagne per week ....

Measures of spirits /liqueurs per week ....

Total: ....

Rating	Units of alcohol/week
A Healthy	7
B Safe	14
C Marginal	21
D Moderate risk	28
E Problematic	35
F Grave risk	50
G Dangerous	63

4 RESULT (Units of acohol per week)

RATING

5 Nutrition

Now for your nutrition. Please answer honestly:
Use the key below to answer the following statements.

10 – true / always	4 – occasionally
8 – almost always	2 – rarely
6 – sometimes	0 – false / never

Enter score here

1 I take time to enjoy every meal

2 I pay attention to both the quality and
quantity of food that I eat

3 I enjoy my food in general and sensible eating
is not a constant battle of willpower

4 I understand the role of my metabolism in my weight
control

5 I am aware of the connection between what I eat and drink
and my overall health

6 I am aware of the connection between what and how I eat
and my performance and energy levels

7 I avoid dieting, preferring to look at the underlying cause if
my weight becomes a problem

8 Complex carbohydrates (bread, rice, pasta, potatoes)
make up at least half of my daily calorie intake

9 I eat a wide variety of foods including vegetables, fresh
fruit, grains and nuts

10 I tend to snack on healthy snacks like fresh fruit, vegetables
or dried fruit

11 I understand the link between my fat intake and my blood
cholesterol levels

12 I avoid eating calorie dense snacks like sweets, cakes and
fried hors d'oeuvres

13 I have control of my sweet tooth
(chocolate, table sugar, pastries, sweet snacks)

14 I am generally active after meals and avoid
sitting and sleeping

15 I eat my last meal more than one hour
before going to bed

16 When travelling I tend to avoid the standard meals offered
on airplanes, boats and trains

17 Even when away on trips I eat healthy balanced meals

18 I drink at least 5 to 8 glasses of pure water daily

19 I do not suffer from constipation or other digestive
troubles

I try to minimize my use of the following:

20 alcohol

21 full fat milk

22 coffee, tea and
caffeine-containing
fizzy drinks

23 eggs

24 salt

25 chocolate

26 refined sugar (table
sugar, ice cream)

27 saturated fat (cheese,
butter, animal fats)

28 fatty meats and skin
(beef, pork, duck)

29 fried foods
(chips, meats, eggs)

30 organ meats
(liver, giblets)

5 TOTAL .... **DIVIDE BY 30 FOR SCORE** ....

Turn over for rating

Rating Nutrition	Questionnaire score
A Optimal	10
B Superior	8
C Average	6
D Below average	3
E Marginal	2
F Poor	0

5 TOTAL ....

RATING ....

> ## Do take the trouble to list your scores and ratings
>
> *The control chart is on the opposite page. You will be quite surprised at the difference when you come to answer exactly the same questions six months into your new health regime.*
>
> *Of course your medical testing cannot alter much but the rest should improve dramatically.*

Two to go. Let's now look at your activity rating:

6 Activity survey

Please use the key below to answer the following statements:

10 – true / always	*4 – occasionally*
8 – almost always	*2 – rarely*
6 – sometimes	*0 – false / never*

Enter score here

☐ 1 I participate in physical exercise more than twice a week

☐ 2 Social and family commitments do not limit my chances to exercise

☐ 3 I regularly vary my exercise activities

☐ 4 I find that exercise can re-energize me if I am tired

☐ 5 I am not overly competitive or obsessive about my participation in physical activity and do not get unduly stressed if I missed a planned session of sport

☐ 6 I recognize the helpfulness of exercise to compensate for the excesses of business life and that activity is critical to my success

☐ 7 Physical activity is written into my weekly agenda

☐ 8 I sleep better when I exercise regularly

☐ 9 Physical activity is an integral part of my stress management strategy

☐ 10 I endeavour to take stairs instead of the lift, walk up and down the escalator and stand in preference to sitting on public transport

6 TOTAL .... **DIVIDE BY 10 FOR SCORE** ....

Rating Nutrition	Questionnaire score
A Outstanding	10
B Superior	9
C Above average	8
D Average	7
E Below average	5
F Fair	4
G Poor	2

RATING ....

7 Stress survey

Please use the key below to answer the following statements.

10 – *true / always*	4 – *occasionally*
8 – *almost always*	2 – *rarely*
6 – *sometimes*	0 – *false / never*

Enter score here

☐ 1 I manage my time well without running short or feeling stressed by my obligations

☐ 2 I make enough time for my personal interests including physical activity

☐ 3 Temper is not a problem for me

☐ 4 Most of my stress is self imposed and I decide how stressed I will be

☐ 5 I recognize how I experience stress and I know when and where to get help

☐ 6 I can pro-actively face a problem (at work and at home) and evaluate what aspects I can and cannot control

☐ 7 I can learn to live with those things I cannot change

☐ 8 I do not have the kind of expectations that set me up for profound disappointment

☐ 9 I get love and affection from people who are important to me

☐ 10 In general I feel very happy about the way life has worked out for me

7 TOTAL .... **DIVIDE BY 10 FOR SCORE** ....

Rating Stress		Questionnaire score
A	Outstanding	10
B	Well managed	8
C	Above average	7
D	Average	5
E	Below average	3
F	Poor	0

RATING ....

RESULTS AND RATINGS

	Test 1 date		Test 2 date		Test 3 date	
	RESULT	RATING	RESULT	RATING	RESULT	RATING
1 Resting Heart Rate (beats/min)						
2 Medical History						
3 Tobacco Use (cigarettes/day)						
4 Alcohol Use (drinks/week)						
5 Nutrition Survey						
6 Activity Survey						
7 Stress Survey						

FITNESS TESTS

If you enjoyed that lifestyle questionnaire, why not try all our fitness tests. There is a control chart (see p. 139), with three columns so you can check your improvement during the year:

Here are the tests you should undertake. The first two, blood pressure and cholesterol limits, will need to come from a doctor but the others can be all self-measured.

The fundamental four (1 to 4)

The first four parameters constitute the four most fundamental health related tests that you will need to carry out. A method for measuring your body fat yourself has been included on the page opposite, however it is only approximate.

1 Blood pressure   a Systolic ....

            b Diastolic ....

Rating systolic blood pressure	Test result mmHG
A *Normal SBP*	135
B *Borderline SBP*	145
C *Severe SBP*	185
D *Dangerous SBP*	260

1a RESULT .... RATING ....

Rating dyastolic blood pressure	Test result mmHG
A *Normal DBP*	85
B *Borderline DBP*	95
C *Severe DBP*	110
D *Dangerous DBP*	140

1b RESULT .... RATING ....

2 Cholesterol   a Total cholesterol ....

            b HDL cholesterol ....

            c TC/HDL ratio ....

Rating Total cholesterol	Test result
A *Very low (ideal)*	2.0
B *Low*	3.0
C *Normal*	4.0
D *Moderate*	5.0
E *High dangerous*	6.5

2a RESULT .... RATING ....

Rating HDL cholesterol	Test result
A *High (ideal)*	1.08
B *Moderate*	0.75
C *Normal*	0.5
D *Low*	0.45
E *Very low (increased risk)*	0.35

2b RESULT .... RATING ....

Rating TC/HDL ratio	Test result
A *Ideal ratio*	2
B *Optimal ratio*	3.4
C *Average ratio*	4.5
D *Marginal ratio*	7
E *Dangerous ratio*	15

2c RESULT .... RATING ....

3 Body fat % of body weight can be estimated using the following guidelines:

Females: Using a tape measure, measure your:

1 Abdomen ($\frac{1}{2}$ inch above the navel)

2 Right thigh (just below the buttocks)

3 Right calf (the widest part,
   halfway between the ankle and knee).

Abdomen	Constant	Right thigh	Constant	Right calf	Constant
25"	30	14"	17	10"	14
26"	31	15"	19	11"	16
27"	32	16"	20	12"	17
28"	33	17"	21	13"	19
29"	34	18"	22	14"	20
30"	36	19"	23	15"	22
31"	37	20"	24	16"	23
32"	38	21"	26	17"	25
33"	39	22"	27	18"	26
34"	40	23"	28	19"	27
35"	42	24"	29	20"	29
36"	43	25"	31	21"	30
37"	44	26"	32	22"	32

Find the constant for each measurement and insert into the following equation:

Example

(29" Abdomen)	34 (constant)
(22" Thigh)	+27 (constant)
Subtotal	61
(14$\frac{1}{2}$" Calf)	−21 (constant)
Subtotal	40
	−21
Approximate Body Fat	**19 %**

Your Results ....

Males: With your tape measure, measure your:

1. Buttocks (maximum protrudence with your heels together)

2 Abdomen ($\frac{1}{2}$" above the navel)

3 Right forearm
   (the widest part, between the elbow and wrist)

Buttocks	Constant	Abdomen	Constant	Right forearm	Constant
28"	29	26"	23	7"	21
29"	30	27"	24	8"	24
30"	31	28"	25	9"	27
31"	32	29"	26	10"	30
32"	34	30"	27	11"	33
33"	35	31"	28	12"	36
34"	36	32"	29	13"	39
35"	37	33"	30	14"	42
36"	38	34"	30	15"	45
37"	39	35"	31	16"	48
38"	40	36"	32	17"	51
39"	41	37"	33	18"	54
40"	42	38"	34		

Find the constant for each measurement and insert into the following equation:

Example

(38" Buttocks)	40 (constant)
(34" Abdomen)	+30 (constant)
Subtotal	70
(8" R.forearm)	−24 (constant)
Subtotal	46
	−19
Approximate Body Fat	**27 %**

Your Results ....

Turn over for rating

Rating Body fat percentage	Age Range					
	18–25	26–35	36–45	46–55	56–65	66–99
A Very lean	7	12	14	16	18	18
B Lean	10	15	18	20	21	21
C Leaner than average	13	18	21	23	24	23
D Average	16	21	24	25	26	25
E Fatter than average	20	24	26	28	28	27
F Over fat	26	28	29	31	31	30
G Markedly over fat	37	37	38	38	38	38

3 RESULT percentage .... RATING...................................

4 Cardio-Fitness Test (beats per minute)

Cardio-vascular efficiency

Find a bench or step approximately 30cm high. Step on and off the bench at a rate of 24 steps per minute for three minutes. Change your leading leg after 1½ minutes to avoid fatigue. When three minutes are up sit down, locate your pulse (either on your wrist or neck – whichever you find easiest) and count every heart beat for a full minute. Counting should commence within 5 seconds of the end of the test. Record the number of beats counted.

Rating Cardio-fitness test	Age Range					
	18–25	26–35	36–45	46–55	56–65	66–99
A Outstanding	65	65	70	75	80	85
B Superior	75	75	80	85	90	95
C Above average	90	90	95	100	105	110
D Average	105	105	110	115	120	125
E Below average	125	125	130	135	140	145
F Fair	150	150	155	160	165	170
G Poor	180	180	185	185	185	185

4 RESULT beats per minute .... RATING ....

5 Weight (kg) ....

6 Height (metres) ....

7 Waist (cm)

Using a tape measure, measure around the level of the navel.

....

8 Hips (cm)

Using a tape measure, measure around the widest protrudence of the buttocks. Work out your waist-to-hip ratio as demonstrated in the results table.

....

Rating Waist to hip ratio	Test result
A Optimal ratio	0.95
B Borderline ratio	0.99
C Android 'apple' ratio	1.40

7 and **8** RATING ....

9 Push-ups (per minute)

Males: with your arms straight and shoulder-width apart bend your elbows, keeping your knees and hips straight throughout, lowering your body until your rib cage is approximately 10cm from the floor (you may wish to use some kind of marker block to touch your chest each time you lower). Then straighten your arms and return to the start position. Count one. Perform as many push-ups as you can in one complete minute. Rests may be taken as often and for as long as is felt necessary and in any position.

Females: keeping your hips, upper thighs and body in a straight line, place your knees on the floor to help support your body weight and lift your feet into the air. Then follow the instructions for males.

Rating Push-ups per minute		Age Range				
	15–19	20–29	30–39	40–49	50–59	60–69
A Outstanding	75	85	85	80	70	60
B Superior	55	65	65	60	50	40
C Above average	35	45	40	40	30	15
D Average	20	30	25	25	15	8
E Below average	15	20	15	15	10	6
F Fair	10	10	10	10	8	5
G Poor	5	5	5	5	5	3

9 RESULT push-ups per minute.......................... RATING ....

10 Abdominal curl-ups (per minute)

Lie on the floor (you may wish to use a mat to protect your back) with your knees bent and feet flat on the floor. Your arms should lie on the floor by your sides. Slowly raise your head, shoulders and upper torso up and forwards off the floor, sliding your fingers forwards along the floor as you do so; your lower back must remain flat on the floor at all times. Mark the furthest point reached by your fingers with anything that can't be easily moved.

Perform as many curl-ups as you can for one complete minute. One curl-up can be counted each time both sets of fingers touch the set mark. Rests can be taken as often and for as long as is felt necessary.

Rating Abdominal curl-ups per minute		Age Range				
	15–19	20–29	30–39	40–49	50–59	60–69
A Outstanding	80	90	90	85	80	65
B Superior	65	75	75	70	65	50
C Above average	40	50	50	45	40	35
D Average	25	35	35	30	25	20
E Below average	15	25	25	20	15	10
F Fair	8	15	15	10	10	8
G Poor	5	5	5	5	5	5

10 RESULT abdominal curl-ups per minute .... RATING ....

11 Squat-jumps (per minute)

Stand sideways on to a wall, reach up with your inside arm (keep your feet flat on the floor) and make a mark. Make a second mark 1 inch above that. To start bend your knees and touch the floor with both sets of fingers, then jump up and touch the wall above the second mark. Count one. Perform as many squat-jumps as you can in one complete minute.

Rating Squat-jumps per minute		Age Range			
	15–29	30–39	40–49	50–59	60–69
A Outstanding	80	75	70	65	60
B Superior	60	55	50	45	40
C Above average	50	45	40	35	30
D Average	35	30	25	20	15
E Below average	25	20	15	10	10
F Fair	20	15	10	8	8
G Poor	15	10	8	5	5

11 RESULT squat-jumps per minute.......................... RATING ....

Rating Wall sit	Seconds completed
A Outstanding	240
B Superior	190
C Above average	150
D Average	110
E Below average	90
F Fair	60
G Poor	30

12 RESULT seconds completed .... RATING ....

Rating Flexibility – cm stretched	Age Range					
	15–19	20–29	30–39	40–49	50–59	60–69
A Outstanding	50	50	50	45	40	35
B Superior	35	35	35	30	25	20
C Above average	30	30	30	25	20	15
D Average	20	20	20	15	10	10
E Below average	15	15	15	10	8	8
F Fair	10	10	10	8	6	4
G Poor	5	5	5	4	3	2

13 RESULT cm stretched .... RATING ....

Rating Reaction	Distance on ruler – cm
A Outstanding	5
B Superior	10
C Above average	15
D Average	25
E Below average	35
F Fair	45
G Poor	50

14 RESULT distance on ruler – cm .... RATING ....

12 Wall sit (seconds)

Stand with your back flat against a wall, feet shoulder width apart. Walk your feet away from the wall, sliding your back down until your knees are bent to approximately 90 degrees and cross your arms over your chest. Hold that position for as long as you can. Record the number of seconds the position was held.

13 Flexibility (cm)

Lie a long ruler or tape measure straight out on the floor. Then sit on the floor with your legs straight out in front of you either side of the tape. The heels of your feet should be placed at the 25cm mark. Keeping your knees straight and flat on the floor, slowly lean forward from the hip and reach out as far along the tape with both hands as you can. Record your maximum reach.

14 Reaction (cm)

You will need the help of a partner for this test, plus two wood, plastic, or metal 50cm rulers and a table. Rest your forearms on the table shoulder-width apart, with your wrists over the edge of the table. Have your partner hold a ruler in each hand vertically with the 'zero' end between your thumb and forefinger. Your partner will then drop one of the rulers which you must catch between your thumb and fingers; measure how far up the ruler you managed to catch it. Take your best score from four random drops and record it.

15 BMI index

Divide weight by height squared.

ASSESSMENT RESULTS TABLE

PARAMETER	TEST 1 DATE		TEST 2 DATE		TEST 3 DATE	
	RESULT	RATING	RESULT	RATING	RESULT	RATING
1a Systolic Blood Pressure (mmHG)						
1b Diastolic Blood Pressure (mmHG)						
2a Total Cholesterol (mmol/L)						
2b HDL Cholesterol (mmol/L)						
2c (TC/HDL Ratio)						
3 Body Fat Percentage						
4 Cardio-Fitness Test (beats per minute)						
5 Weight (kg)						
6 Waist (cm)						
7 Hip (cm)						
8 Waist/Hip Ratio (waist ÷ by hip)						
9 Push-ups (per minute)						
10 Curl-ups (per minute)						
11 Squat-jumps (per minute)						
12 Wall Sit (seconds)						
13 Flexibility (cm)						
14 Reaction (cm)						
15 BMI body weight (÷ square of height)						

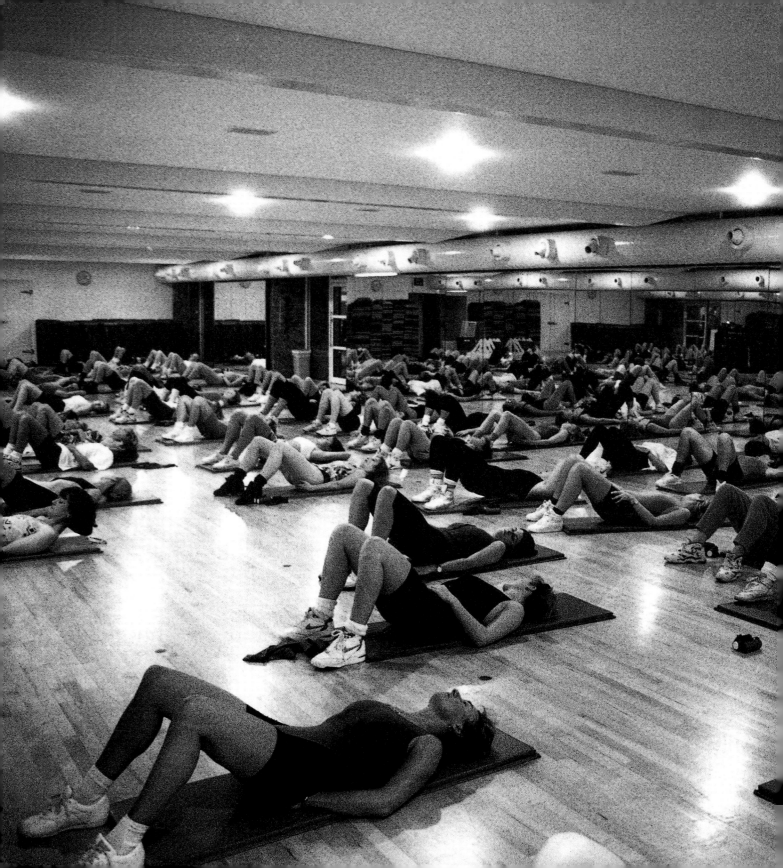

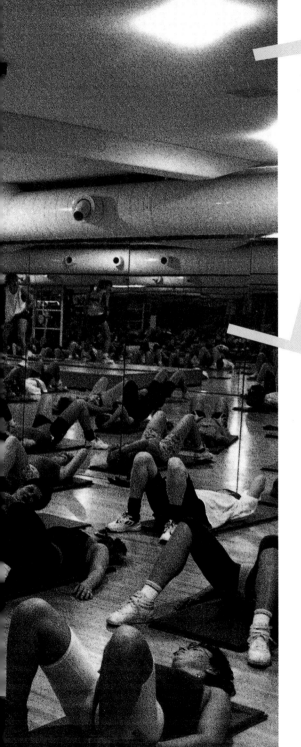

CHAPTER TEN

DOING IT SLOW AND EASY

There is no magic formula to becoming fit and healthy. It is not like winning a lottery – one day you are poor and struggling, then, magically, you buy the right ticket and you are rich. Attaining fitness just does not work like that.

Nor can any amount of wishing and dreaming make the difference. You have to do it yourself. A positive decision must be reached, a plan conceived, time allotted and action taken. Depending upon how unfit you are to start with there could be some immediate effects. If so, you begin to feel better within a few days – after a week or two you start to feel marvellous. But around a month or so into the programme the danger period starts. Boredom can begin to take over. You can begin to feel that the regular exercise, and taking all that care with your food, is becoming tedious. You forget how you used to feel. You begin to miss one or two exercise sessions because 'you are really too busy', and you start to take more frequent liberties with your food.

> *You forget how you used to feel. You begin to miss one or two exercise sessions because 'you are really too busy'*

What happens next is that the occasional missed exercise session becomes the norm and because you still feel okay, and you have not put on that much weight, you do not worry too much about it all until, suddenly, you have completed a four-month circle back to where you were when you first resolved to get fitter and look after your health more.

The only thing is that since you have already tried and failed, you will find it hard to get as enthusiastic again next time you get the yen. It is a lot easier living without regular exercise and eating whatever and whenever you like ... except once again you are susceptible to all the problems of physical inactivity – general lethargy, frequent minor illnesses, and a tendency to obesity; you are also running a much higher risk of heart disease or cancer.

This is the trap beginning exercisers must guard against.

Ironically it is often those who start the most enthusiastically who begin to waiver the earliest.

Resume exercise slowly. Make it easy. Do not rush and sacrifice, but rather try and find a regular time you can fit into each day. Soon it will be that part of the day you treasure the most. I kid you not.

Routine makes life easier

If you have developed a routine at the office or when you do the housework you will no doubt know how much easier it all becomes when your day is organized into segments.

An occasional change may feel like a holiday but getting back to the routine is a welcome relief and you feel that much more efficient again. So it is with exercise. Certainly it can be kept interesting by varying sites, types, exertion levels and/or companions, but if you maintain the timetable (each morning or lunch time, or on the way home, or whenever) you will find it that much easier to sustain.

Keeping to the correct foods should be easy, too, if you remind yourself just how poisonous things like chocolate bars, potato crisps or sweet biscuits really are. Your occasional splurge should at least be directed to foods with some worthwhile nutrients. You need to eliminate completely those with high sugar, salt, refined flour or fat content.

Taking it easy

If you can determine that you will exercise each day and then, on the rare occasions that becomes impossible (and it will), never to miss more than 48 hours no matter what comes up, you will find that soon your body will make it easy for you and demand to have its workout. Fitness becomes a sort of daily drug you cannot do without. That feeling, dear reader, is sheer joy. You feel just terrific. On the way to that sort of Utopia, you should ensure that no session is too tough. As we have stressed, getting fit takes time.

In fact for the first three or four months, you train mainly in order to be able to train a little harder in the next session.

No one can build anything without solid foundations. The first six months, or if you are really serious, two years, of training is purely foundation. Remember it is your life we are now talking about. As the height of the building (the quality and length of your life) is indeterminable – all you know is that you want it to go as high, and last as long, as you can make it – the base has to be as strong and as solid as possible. Essentially, it has to be solid enough, and strong enough to support all your aspirations for a long, active lifestyle.

There is no hurry. Nothing worthwhile was built quickly. Begin with a few minutes for each exercise and gradually, ever so slowly, build up from there. Never be so tired from one day's training that you cannot repeat it, should you so wish, the next day, and the next and the next.

You should feel okay, a little tired perhaps but fine nevertheless, whenever you complete a workout. After a shower and a little rest you should be even better. Certainly, with no exceptions, you should be feeling better after an exercise session then you did before it, otherwise it has been too hard a workout and you will need to tone down the next one slightly. I liken it to getting a deep sun tan. Go out in the sun for too long, too soon and the result is sunburn. But take it easily, just a few minutes or so to start, gradually increasing the time each day, and the result is a great tan. Miss a few days and you have to go back to the start. Exercising is exactly the same. Too much, too soon and you are just burning yourself out. Take it step by step, build up slowly and there is no limit to your improvement.

Whenever you do specific exercises they too should be undertaken slowly and under control. Actually they are more difficult when performed in this way. And much more beneficial.

Rush any exercise and you only truly work the accelerating muscles in that particular movement; the balance of it is achieved through momentum.

Weightlifters thrust to maximize the weight they are lifting in comparison to their strength. They rely on the speed of the push. If they were forced to lift the weight more slowly, the weights being lifted would be reduced by 20% or more.

If you want to stretch a muscle you do so slowly and then hold. If you jerked it, you could do damage by taking it past its present limit and out of control. Similar concerns should dictate your movements when lifting weights or undertaking any exercises – do them slowly to gain the maximum benefit. Keep control.

What about losing speed? and injuries?

Stronger muscles are never slower muscles. Speed is inherited through the genes generally and then honed by technique and specific reaction training. But the fitter and stronger you get from your slow controlled-strength workouts the more able will these same muscles be when coping with sudden movements.

As for injuries, I had a career extending over ten years, racing throughout the year on the road, cross country and all sorts of track, week in and week out – 60 to 70 races a year.

This was combined with a training programme totalling more than 100 miles weekly. Yet I did not get injured. Now, 30 years later, I have never suffered the joint and muscle problems which more often than not plague ex-sportsmen.

I firmly believe I have avoided these repercussions, despite intense training and competition, through proper nutrition, adequate rest and, most importantly, consistent strength workouts.

Too many sports people of all denominations ignore their need for supplementary and complementary weight training to strengthen their joints, muscles and tendons. Ironically they use the same excuse as the layman for not exercising at all – they 'haven't the time'. In most cases they are too busy practising their 'skills', or 'too tired' from their other training.

The only reason they have not got the time is the same as it is with everybody else: they just have not organized their day properly.

Everybody has the time. The no time excuse is camouflage for 'I do not really want to do it'.

It has always astounded me how sensible athletes will spend hours each day for years developing fitness and skills, while risking breakdowns at crucial times because they are not going that one step further and protecting themselves with proper supplementary workouts.

It is their insurance, and who would spend years building a house without taking out insurance so that, when it is finished, it will not fall down or be burnt out before you get the chance to live in it.

> *The no time excuse is camouflage for 'I do not really want to do it'*

> *It is our job, as adults, to allow children to develop – but within the safety limits which we can provide*

Too old? Too young?

You can never be too old to start an exercise programme. Or too fat or too thin or too anything. The type of programme you undertake has to be structured to fit your particular state of health or fitness, physical limitations and lifestyle circumstances. And you can do it by beginning slowly and regularly undertaking any of the exercise routines we have outlined in this book. If you have to adapt it to make it simpler at first then go to it. But be regular, do it daily, establish a routine, and most of all stick to it.

During my youth there used to be an advertisement on Australian radio for a fly spray which continually urged its audience 'when you're on to a good thing, stick to it'. Very basic advice but very pertinent when referring to an exercise programme.

Too young? Heavens no. There is no reason why youngsters cannot exercise for two or three hours, or even more, a day. We did, but back then it was called play. If we were inside for more than 30 minutes, our parents would shunt us out into the yard or street to play some more.

From the time I was four I walked or ran the mile to school, and back, rode bicycles around and around the block, played football or running games like 'chase', 'rounders' or 'release'. Girls rode, skipped, hopped and played too. Had people thought we were exercising I suppose they would have said we were doing too much. It did not seem peculiar to me, up to the age of sixteen, when I graduated from high school, to run and play football and generally 'work out' two or three times daily for a total of three to four hours. It was perfectly normal. No one was ever too tired from it. Yet, after leaving school and actually beginning to train with a local football team, I was told that if I practised or worked out more than twice weekly I would go 'stale'. What nonsense, but that was the theory then, and it is not so different today among footballers. I firmly believe the amount and type of exercise to which a youngster up to seven

years of age is exposed will determine what sort of an athlete he or she becomes later in life ('Give me the boy until he is seven and I shall give the man' is an old Jesuit saying which is very true). Further than that, frequent enjoyable 'exer-play' at a young age influences the whole future attitude towards health and fitness in children.

If parents do not exercise themselves, if they feel the children are 'safer' inside watching television or playing computer games, then forget it. By the time the kids are seven they will so lack co-ordination that playing any sport, or undertaking any physical activity, will be an embarrassment; they will be awkward, feel uncomfortable and attract derision/laughter when, or if, they ever do try. No child will persist in these circumstances. They will grow up ignorant of the joys of nature, health and exercise unless some dramatic turnaround in their lifestyle takes place.

So yes, encourage the young. If you can play with them yourself so much the better – walking, ball games, tennis, hopscotch (if you are still able), and whatever game they like. Also try to help them develop their climbing, balancing and co-ordinative skills by providing safe challenges for them. Kids naturally are both cautious and adventurous. They will try something new but are usually very wary of going too far too soon. Nature has naturally given them the instinct for survival. It is our job to allow them to develop – but within the safety limits which we can provide.

For example, let them climb but be certain there is a cushioned mat to fall on. Let them balance but be ready to support them if they totter, and so on. No one gains in strength, co-ordination and physical and mental ability more quickly than a young child given a free rein in his or her environment.

Instead of limiting them our task should be guide and protect them whilst allowing them their freedom. Easier said than done, I know, and another field in which government have been noticeably lacking in appreciation and assistance.

No one should be surprised if the kids of today, allowed to grow into teenagers without the stimulation of a healthy environment, become the young troublemakers of tomorrow.

The government spend millions treating these problems after they occur. How much simpler it would be to go to the cause and spend more time and attention providing proper environments to ensure pre-teens mature healthily.

Tumble Tots

In fact, in the early days of Cannons in 1984, we launched a national concept for youngsters up to seven years of age called Tumble Tots.

It came about through my enthusiasm for keeping toddlers physically active during their early years. I have many friends who are primary school teachers and they often described to me the huge diversity in basic motor and ball skills of seven- to ten-year-olds in their schools. Of course, those who feel inept are often exasperated through the years as they do not like to expose their lack of ability in front of their classmates. They avoid ball games or physical education (often aided and abetted by parents who don't like to see their children 'embarrassed').

This problem has always been there but has worsened considerably over the past few years with the publicity given to unsupervised children being kidnapped or assaulted. Letting the kids loose in the park is not the option it once was.

I was looking for a way in which Cannons could be involved with pre-school children's physical development when the efforts of a renowned gymnasium coach in Southampton was brought to my attention. While headquartered there as the regional director, Bill Cosgrave had built up a successful programme for babies of a few months right through to children of five years old. He had called it 'Tumble Tots' but did not have the financial wherewithal to launch the programme on a wider scale.

So we purchased his fledgling company, retained Bill and his wife Jenny as consultants, together with their friend Nik Stuart, possibly Britain's greatest ever Olympic gymnast, added some investment funds and set up a country-wide marketing organization.

The idea is for interested and qualified people to purchase licences for particular areas. We supply portable gymnastic equipment and special trailers, and they hire halls around their district and retain assistants so that they can operate 60-minute-long classes for the various age groups. The youngsters are divided into four small groups and are moved in their groups from station to station, each 'station' concentrating on a particular movement or activity. During the session at these 'stations' they balance, climb, practise ball skills, undertake flexibility and tumbling exercises – all disguised as play.

Tumble Tots builds social interchange (getting on with other kids), discipline (staying in their groups) and most importantly the confidence of getting to know their own physical capabilities.

If you walk through a park with youngsters, their natural instinct is to run, hop, climb, or zig-zag. This is nature working, developing naturally, through their own instincts, their physical and mental capabilities at a faster rate than they will ever be able to replicate in their later years. These are, without doubt, the most important years in human development (as I keep repeating). This is when parents have to be prepared to put in the time, especially nowadays.

Physically, any adult should have more stamina then a five- to ten-year-old child – but let us see who tires first! Your children may be able to teach you a thing or two about physical activity, and about the quiet enjoyment of the simple things in life such as the sun, trees and gardens, the seashore and the environment, companionship and, perhaps, life's priorities.

> *Your children may be able to teach you a thing or two about physical activity*

> *No one gains in strength, co-ordination and physical or mental ability more quickly than a young child given a free rein in his or her environment*

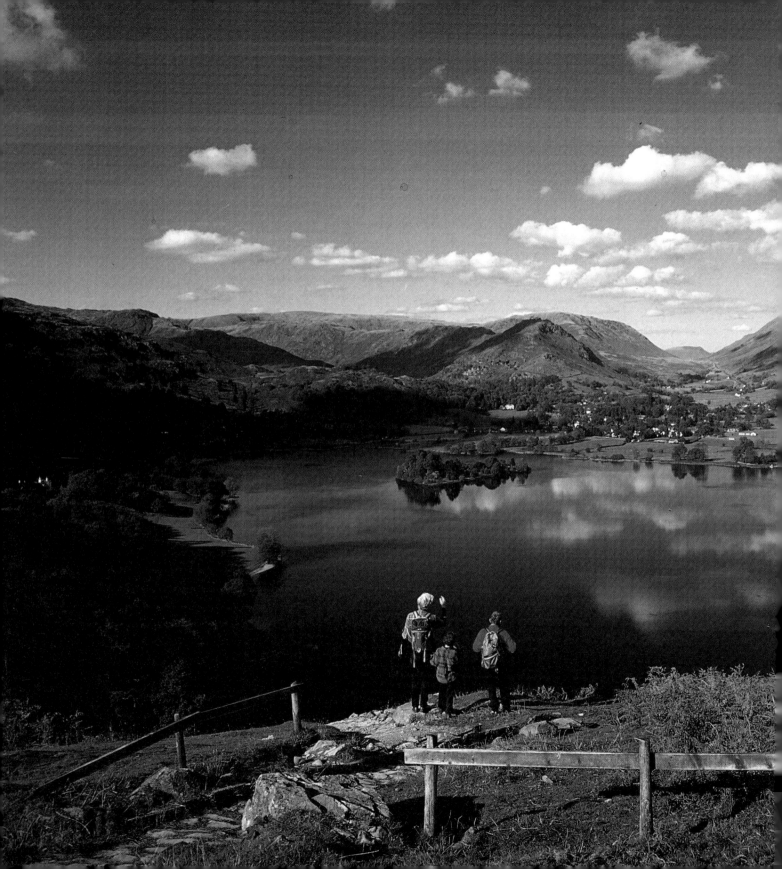

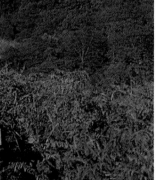

CHAPTER ELEVEN

DIFFERENT WAYS OF GOING ABOUT IT

Certainly the basis of improved health and fitness depends upon the quality and regularity of your workouts and your success in balancing and limiting your nutritional intake.

But these are the routine. Actually playing sport or participating in some sort of outdoor activity can provide a whole well of extra enjoyment.

Most active people know all about sports such as golf, tennis, rugby, football, hockey, squash, etc. – sports regularly played and which provide weekends of fun and enjoyment for tens of thousands. However there are many other ways to enjoy activities out-of-doors not nearly as well known and so we have asked some of our consultants to talk about their particular interests.

The first of these 'volunteers' is Felicity Butler, the UK women's climbing champion. Felicity has been

There are many other ways to enjoy activities out-of-doors...

associated with us for a couple of years now, advising and helping our members at Cannons on using our indoor climbing treadmill which adds an extra dimension of difficulty and challenge to a number of their workouts. She tells of the joys of climbing. But not on arduous and dangerous mountain slopes with expensive expeditions. Rather Felicity specializes in climbing the boulders and rock walls around the country available to all with the inclination and the nerve.

Then John Coster and his team (John is principal of 'World Adventure Consultants') give us a few brief notes on some of the other options open to you. If any of these appeal, contact him in the UK on 081 981 9849 and he can tell you how you can participate in and explore any of these pursuits. Over the years his firm has been responsible for organizing groups of our members to join him in all types of adventure weeks and weekends.

Feeding a passion – Felicity Butler

'Climbing is a hobby; a sport; a passion; for some, a way of life; and for professional climbers, it *becomes* their life. It is an activity difficult to define but which inspires admiration, curiosity and bewilderment in the casual onlooker. I became a full-time climber in 1991, and today, in 1994, I make a modest living from it. As a professional climber I am often asked what is the biggest mountain I have scaled. People wonder how I manage to carry all the mountaineering equipment necessary to tackle those formidable snow- and glassy ice-laden peaks. They marvel at how brave (or foolish) I am and shiver at the thought of the cold and discomfort of a mountain bivouac.

I take a deep breath and explain that I am a *rock climber*; interested in climbing demanding routes up crags and cliffs, usually no more than 100 feet or so high ... and then coming down to the bottom (perhaps along a path or lowering off a point) and then climbing another route. This invariably leaves the bemused enquirer with the inevitable question, 'Why?'

> **Unlike athletics and gymnastics, climbing requires a partnership in which there has to be total trust**

Defining climbing is like trying to define athletics. It has many facets but, unlike athletics, its various activities merge into one another. Mountain climbers who aspire to reach the tops of big mountains often find themselves tackling steep rock faces, and rock climbers may choose to climb a long rock route which takes them to the top of a mountain. At the other end of the spectrum, climbers – far from wanting to reach the top of a mountain or cliff – may only aspire to mastery of a few hard moves on a boulder.

Called 'bouldering', this type of climbing is very short and needs no ropes. The movements are technical and physically demanding and more akin to gymnastics where strength, co-ordination and agility are of the essence.

Unlike athletics and gymnastics, however, climbing requires a partnership of generally two, in which there has to be total trust since inattention could result in serious injury. The leader climbs up on the 'sharp end' of the rope and places protection in case of a fall. The partner belays, holding the rope to arrest a fall and playing the rope out as the leader climbs. These roles are frequently alternated between partners as they take it in turns to lead.

As climbers, we often see each other in nerve-racking situations, exposing our weaknesses and strengths. It is this camaraderie of climbing, the sharing of difficult situations as well as the intense emotions that climbing evokes, which lodges most deeply in the memory of a good day out.

In Britain, there are a great number of different types of rock, providing very interesting and varied climbing, often in areas both beautiful and wild. To appreciate the whole spectrum of British climbing it is necessary to travel a fair bit. But being a member of a local climbing club makes this much easier as climbers can share cars and expenses. For most people, climbing is a hobby – brief periods of excitement to intersperse the routine or stress of their working lives. Climbing as a hobby was, for me, like a valium panacea, its effect spanning the whole week. First, the anticipation of the weekend with the planning of a venue and the routes to climb. And, then, away from my work and the city, the intense concentration of physical and mental powers needed to scale and climb removed all thoughts and worries from my mind. Only the few metres of rock surrounding me were important; the holds I was striving to reach, together with the necessity of placing traditional protection of nuts and friends in small cracks in the rock, were my only concern.

Climbing can be so engrossing that an hour or more may feel like a few minutes only. Sometimes reaching the top gives rewards of stunning views far from the madding crowds, but there are always feelings of elation and satisfaction for achieving a hard-won goal, of winning a battle with nature and yourself. One long climb of several rope lengths may take the whole day, but then the other serious activity of climbers can begin – in the pub with tales and reminiscences over a bevy or two.

In this respect, climbing creates an invariably lively social forum, drawing people together from all walks of life. When there is no other obvious common ground between fellow climbers, there is always climbing … winter, summer, mountains, sea cliffs, crags, adventure climbing, sports climbing, nuts, bolts, friends … there is never a shortage of topics.

In Britain, there is a strong following of traditional *'adventure'* climbing where the protection is carried by the leader and placed on lead. As the second climbs up with the rope taken in from above, he removes the various pieces of equipment. Traditional climbing has the attraction that a climber can, in theory, ascend any piece of rock within his ability without anyone else having been there previously to place in situ protection bolts. Protecting bolted up climbs is very easy and the leader need take only a few short slings, each with two Karabinas attached; one for clipping the bolt and the other to clip the rope through. With less

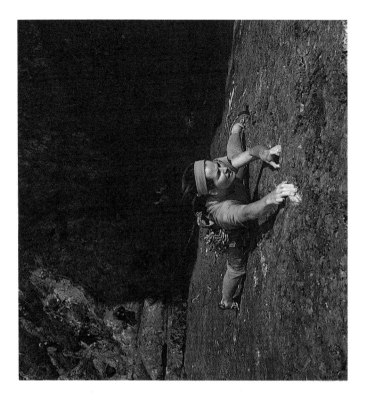

objective danger, climbing on bolts – or *'sports'* climbing – is easier for the lead, although the climbs are usually more difficult physically.

Sports climbers frequently aspire to climbing routes too difficult for them to achieve without falling off several times on the first and, possibly, many subsequent attempts. But, after practising the move sequences, they are eventually able to climb the route in one push. 'Working' routes in this way has produced some very hard climbs indeed, with Britain being home to some of the hardest.

The issue of 'to bolt, or not to bolt' probably causes the most passionate discussions between climbers in Britain but, for the continentals, there is no problem; if you can climb it, bolt it! In some ways, this attitude makes climbing accessible to more people but, in Britain, the bolted crags are limited, with the wilder and more remote sea cliffs and mountain crags remaining traditional.

The co-operation and trusting partnerships necessary in climbing make it hard to comprehend real competition, other than between climber and rock. Of course, friendly competition has always existed, bouldering moves on short problems, for example, and, naturally, there is some rivalry between climbers. However, bolts on climbs have allowed climbing to enter the competitive arena on a worldwide scale. Enormous imposing structures built of scaffolding and resin panels are erected at venues all over the world to which the best climbers from each country travel.

The climbs are set by professional route setters who try to make the routes spectacular and of the right difficulty to separate the climbers' ability. Except for the very best climbers, falling at some stage in the competition is inevitable and there are professional belayers to hold the ropes.

Far from being a relief from stress, competition climbing requires careful mental preparation to turn nervous anticipation into positive energy for the task ahead. The ordeal may seem as hard as any physical challenge ever attempted and yet the excitement draws climbers back to compete again and again, ever striving to improve their world ranking. In the final rounds, the atmosphere is electric as the top climbers take it in turn to pit their strength against a route of extreme difficulty. The competitor who climbs the highest wins the competition, a trophy and cash.

And yet, at the end of it all, true to climbing tradition, all the competitors, coaches, judges, and climbers, relax together in a big party. Even though the venues may be thousands of miles apart the climbers' faces change very little and they are bound in friendship by their mutual obsession.

Although competitive climbing is still a young sport, prize money and sponsorship have given rise to professional sports climbers whose training is as dedicated as for any other professional sport. Sponsorship allows me to train and travel to different climbing areas in Britain and abroad and, in this respect, my sport feeds my climbing passion. Competitions are simply another facet of the climbing 'gem', providing a channel to indulge in other aspects as well.

I can think of only one answer to the big question, 'Why do you climb?' and that is because it is there. All climbers climb because they love to do so; there is rarely any purpose to it. Even the very best competition climbers could earn a better living from a regular fulltime job.

So there is no reason; we climb, therefore we are!

The outdoor alternatives – John Coster

Mountain walking

Mountaineering or mountain climbing is the name given to walking, rock scrambling and climbing activities in the mountains. Walking, in the form of rambling and hiking, is probably the easiest and most popular recreational pursuit. Mountain walking, or fell and hill walking, has over the years become one of the UK's fastest growing leisure activities. It can be adventurous, challenging and exciting. But it can also be very dangerous unless you are well prepared and properly equipped. You have to be aware of the hazards of the mountains.

Although the British mountains are not nearly as high as those in Europe, they should not be treated lightly. The terrain is rough, the weather can change in a matter of minutes, and the distances involved in walking in the mountains are much greater than on the flat. However, if you take the right equipment and use your commonsense it is possible to enjoy the spectacular scenery that exists in these areas of Britain.

Orienteering

Orienteering involves completing a course by finding your way to and between controls, marked on the special map as circles, in the shortest possible time, using cross-country running and map reading skills. The

> *Walking, in the form of rambling and hiking, is probably the easiest and most popular recreational pursuit*

controls are not hidden and are fairly easy to find.

Orienteering is therefore mainly a test of your ability to select the best and quickest route between the controls. This does not always mean sprinting along the shortest distance to the next control, because the shortest distance may take you through very difficult terrain, such as thick forest or up steep slopes. It is often best to take longer but safer routes, such as easy-to-follow paths or tracks where the chances of getting lost and losing time are reduced.

Canoeing

Almost every town has a canoe club or outdoor pursuits centre where water based activities take place. It is one of the few adventurous sports that is truly available to everyone in the country. Britain is amongst the top canoeing nations in the world and the facilities available are improving every year.

The general term canoeing covers a whole collection of different activities:

1 Inland water – rivers, lakes and canals for racing (sprint, wild water, slalom and long distance).
2 Sea – for canoe surfing, sailing and long distance trips.
3 Swimming pool –- canoe polo, training and skills development.

Many people begin canoeing in a swimming pool. Basic safety and paddling skills can be learned in a controlled, clean and warm environment. You will find that canoeing on rivers, lakes, canals or the sea is totally different. In Britain, almost all waterways and the surrounding land are privately owned, making access to the most exciting water very difficult.

Abseiling

Abseiling is the name given to a controlled slide down a rope. It is a very useful technique to learn, enabling you to get down from the top of a rock climb, as well as being an exciting sport in its own right, now having

its own governing body. Guidelines must be followed when setting up an abseiling anchor point; always use a separate safety rope. There are a number of ways to abseil but the most acceptable methods are:

a The classic abseil – the original method using no equipment other than the rope itself, which is passed around the body; this provides the friction to control the descent.
b Using a descendeur – a metal device designed to make abseiling quicker and more comfortable. The safest and easiest to use is the figure-of-eight descendeur.

Mountain biking

The national parks offer the greatest potential for mountain biking in Britain. There are literally hundreds of miles of 'Rights of Way' open to cyclists across summits, passes, forests, moorland and along valleys. The range of challenges is tremendous. There are easy routes that offer peace and tranquillity amongst fine scenery with few technical or navigational problems, and then there are the full-blown mountain bike rides which will test even the most experienced and accomplished riders.

The type of mountain bike you use is of course a highly personal thing but if you are going to take it into real mountain bike country it should be as light as possible, mechanically sound with effective brakes and uncluttered. Tyres need to have at least a two-inch section: a large contact surface area minimizes any damage to soft ground.

Take a basic tool kit and spares with you, but remember you still have to carry it. For clothing, choose from the large range designed for climbers and walkers. Take a combination of clothes which are windproof, waterproof and insulate even when wet. Your footwear should have a good grip, and of course do not forget your helmet.

> " *In Britain, almost all waterways and the surrounding land are privately owned, making access to the most exciting water very difficult* "

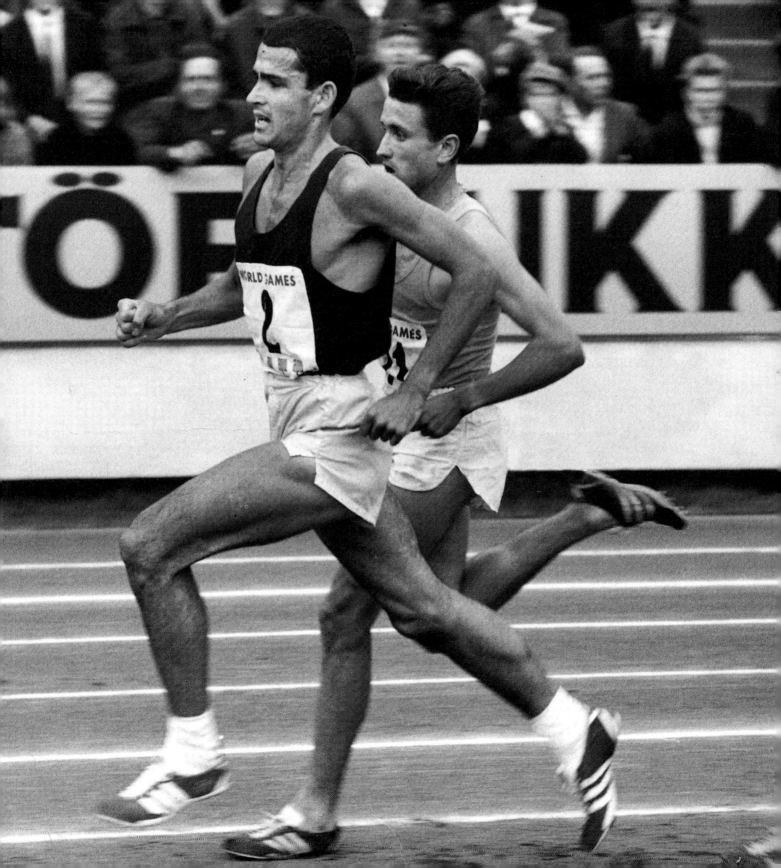

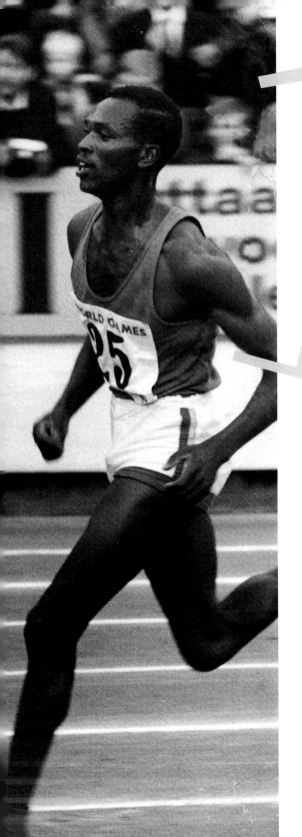

CHAPTER TWELVE

OUR WAY

Why should you believe us? Will what we have told you in this book work for you? To properly answer these questions I must first of all tell you a little about myself.

Right through my life I have been one of those people who always wanted to know what, how, and/or why about everything.

When I started to train seriously for athletics the famous Austrian coach Franz Stampfl convinced me his methods made sense. I did try working out once with the notorious Percy Ceruty only to discover his well-publicized free thinking was a mostly chaotic, illogical mass of irrelevant theory.

Later I found Franz's training schedules too rigid. Although I had no argument with the sound logic of his approach and he was undoubtedly a great inspirer and tactician, I felt there had to be some freer and more enjoyable way to improve performance than undertaking the Stampfl repetition quarters, halves and three-quarters on the track night after night.

The type of training I started to do was much more simplistic; we just ran, usually barefooted, on grass but, importantly, also in the hills each weekend. Later I added the one surging track session each week and we raced in inter-club, cross-country, relays, road races, indoor tracks, outdoor tracks (all types, there was no let up).

> *I felt there had to be some freer and more enjoyable way to improve performance*

> *I understand the aspirations of business people, their day to day problems and the restrictions they experience in fitting in time for exercise*

I was told this was all wrong. That there had to be a start and finish to a season. That I was over-racing, training too slowly, and doing insufficient track work. They told me that this was not what they were doing in the rest of the world, and that it was completely contradictory to current thinking.

All I knew was that I was listening to my own body and instinctively following it. Unless someone could prove absolutely that I was wrong then I would continue to do so, seeing the results I was achieving were pretty good. I thought training should be enjoyable and relatively easy. I wondered why I should copy the Europeans when it was them who I wanted to beat.

The then 10,000 metres record of 28.14.2 was said to be the ultimate. It was supposed to be impossible for anyone to run faster over the distance. And thirteen minutes was reckoned to be just about as quick as anyone would ever run for three miles (the record, at the time, was 13 minutes 10.0 seconds).

Why?

I did not consciously try to break these barriers. In fact I never really set any ultimate target for what I thought I could run. I just wanted to go as fast as I could for as long as possible and see how fast this was. This was considered to be wrong as well. You were supposed to set goals and work towards them. My reasoning was and is:

As soon as you set yourself a goal then you are immediately limiting your thinking and inhibiting your actions.

Either your goal is too high and you are doomed to be disappointed, no matter how well you did, or it is too low, and you really never realize your full potential.

Why not just let it happen by concentrating only on improving each performance, and in getting better week by week. That way you never know at just what level you will finish up. I know that when I started running I did not even dream I was good enough to compete in the Olympics, let alone set new world

records. But one thing led to another. While improving as much as I could from one run to the next, I found suddenly I was breaking through barriers no one (me included) had considered possible. And it all comes about by just taking that one step at a time, never limiting your thinking or considering something is impossible or wrong just because no one has ever done it before.

Whilst travelling and racing I channelled my curiosity into learning as much as I could about how and why the body functions the way it does, and what anyone could do to improve his/her own performance. I studied training for all sorts of sports. Everything was of interest. My conclusions were:

a There are no limits on what the human body can do. The mind and our own imagination are inhibiting factors as much as the type of preparation undertaken.

b You train to prepare your body so that you can get it to go to the very limit of your own particular ability, but it takes time.

c Most of us do not know, nor will we ever train hard enough over a sufficiently long period to discover what we can do *personally*.

Our parameters are set by our own concepts of what is possible and the amount of time we are prepared to dedicate.

How does this relate to you?

Because I am, was and have always been of this mind, I have studied and sorted out the most efficient way of getting fit. Throughout my running career I was first and foremost a business man, training as a chartered accountant and passing all my examinations while working full time in an accountant's office. I mixed with others in all the professions daily for eight to ten hours as my athletic training was always secondary and fitted into my daily routine after hours (the day I set my first world record I worked a normal day in the

PREVIOUS PAGE *This is the way I liked to run - out in front, pushing hard. Here, in the World Games of 1965, I am leading from fellow world record holders Michel Jazy of France and Kipchoge Keino of Kenya.*

office, went to the park and broke it in a twilight meet – the race commenced at 7.00 pm). I think I understand the aspirations of business people, their day to day problems and the restrictions they experience in fitting into their schedules some time for exercise.

Hence when I decided I wanted to be involved with health and fitness on a fulltime basis in 1976 (after retiring from competition in 1970) my aim was to make things simple for people in my sports clubs. I was determined they would not become cathedrals to medical clap-trap and voodoo magic, but remain places which could ensure the users a decent, no non-sense workout, in clean, interesting premises with the best, most effective equipment, developed and assisted by knowledgeable, friendly staff. For about twenty years now this has remained my aim.

What we have put together at Cannons reflects this attitude. Our main aim is to convince people of the merits and advantages of a healthy lifestyle wherever they may decide to work out. We provide the latest equipment, the best premises, the most knowledgable staff and so hope that they will choose us, but that is not as important as persuading them to start looking after themselves with regular sensible exercise.

All our people at Cannons have assisted in completing these writings, especially our consultant medic John Briffa, and indeed most have assisted before now in the evaluation of our principles and practices in the years we have been in the UK.

Do they work?

Of course they work! Our members, both in Australia and in the UK have thrived and the clubs have prospered. There is nothing more satisfying to me than changing someone's lifestyle for the better. Literally thousands have come to us overweight and overstressed, finding it difficult to perform to their ability at the office, or at home.

They discover just how dramatically improved fitness can turn this all around, and immediately

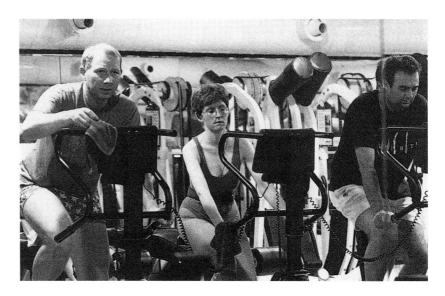

become great disciples of their new lifestyle, enthusiastically relating their personal experiences to their friends. It is all very exciting and worthwhile and, despite my accounting qualifications, I would not want to be in any other business. It is fantastic to experience and watch how much people's personalities and fortunes can alter with a dose of fitness.

Is ours the only way?

Heavens no. There are so many ways to go about it. We think ours is the most direct, and the most effective. But there are no secrets, no one way and, as I have said repeatedly, no magic wand. It all really depends upon you, and how convinced you are of the merits of becoming fit and healthy, and how committed you become.

If you are a believer, and have the dedication, I can promise you that you cannot imagine how well you will feel in six months' time if you start your fitness regime today, and determine to continue daily for at least a period to see just how different you will feel. I guarantee the roses will smell sweeter than you could ever have dreamed.

Believe me, the stakes are high. I wish you well.

It is fantastic to watch how much people's personalities and fortunes can alter with a dose of fitness

PUBLISHER'S NOTE ON RON CLARKE

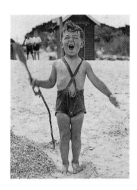

Ron Clarke on a beach

After setting world record times as a junior (under nineteen) for the one mile, two miles, three miles and 5,000m, Ron Clarke virtually retired from athletics in 1956, after completing his National Service, to pursue his business career as a chartered accountant, and establish a family (he and his wife Helen married in 1958 and have three children).

Then, in 1962, Ron made a dramatic re-entry into the sport, winning the Australian Cross-country Championship and surprisingly gaining a silver medal in a class three-mile field in the Perth Commonwealth Games (in his wake were North American champion Bruce Kidd, African champion Kip Keino, European champion Bruce Tulloh and the then world record holder, Alby Thomas).

The next year, after finishing a normal day's work as head office accountant for Lamson Paragon, an international printing group, he walked down to Olympic Park and proceeded to break two world records. One of these, the 10,000m established by Pytor Bolotnikov, was supposed to be untouchable.

Thereafter Ron tore apart the record books, breaking eighteen official world records and a zillion unofficial ones, won three more silver medals at Commonwealth Games, and an Olympic Bronze in 1964 at Tokyo (his most important Olympics, at Mexico City in 1968, at the peak of his form, was ruined for him by the altitude and the advantage this gave to his closest rivals).

He became renowned for competing continuously during four-week forays in Europe, fitting in as many as fifteen top class races in six or seven different countries in the 28 days, zig-zagging back and forth across the continent.

More than any other, Ron Clarke was the pioneer of modern distance runners. He challenged established traditions and medical theories, he raced often and at the highest standard, he broke world records by greater margins than anyone else had ever done before (or since) and he exploded the 'hate your opponent' philosophy as the only way to succeed, as he deliberately sought out and befriended his rivals. Similarly, he proved that the no-pain-no-gain training routines practised at the time were hog-wash, by demonstrating that training could be fun and effective and, as well, be combined with a full-time business career.

If told there were limitations, he asked, 'Why?' When faced with a challenge, it was, 'Why not?' When his business career switched to health and fitness clubs, he determined that their members would benefit, as he had done, from an emphasis on enjoyment and effectiveness. When he took charge of the Cannons Club in 1983, there were 1,000 members and the place was bankrupt. Within six months it was thriving, and now there is no more successful commercially owned club in the world.

We are proud and pleased to have the opportunity to present the inspiring, effective yet simple principles and practices of healthy living – total living, in fact – with Ron and his most able team at Cannons.

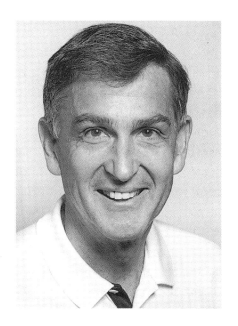

Medals and Records

Set World Bests as Junior: 1 mile, 2 miles, 3 miles and 5,000 metres, 1955
Final Torch Bearer, Olympic Games 1956
Set 18 world track records – all distances from 1-hour run to 2 miles
First athlete to break 13 minutes for 3 miles, and 28 minutes for 10,000 metres
Won 12 Australian Championships and set 36 Australian records
Captain, Australian Olympic team, Olympic Games 1964
Bronze medal, Olympic Games 1964
4 silver medals, Commonwealth Games 1962, 1966, 1970
BBC World Sportsman of the Year, 1965
International Association of Sports Writers, World Sportsman of the Year, 1965
French Academy of Sport World Sportsman of the Year, 1966
AAA Champion of the Year (UK), 1965, 1966, 1967
Australian Sportsman of the Year, 1965, 1966

REFERENCE LIST - Dr John Briffa

Articles

1 Bengtsson C. and others
Association of serum lipid concentrations and obesity with mortality in women: twenty-year follow up of participants in prospective population study in Göteborg, Sweden.
British Medical Journal 1993; 307: 1385–1388

2 Ripsin C. M. and Keenen J. M.
The effects of dietary oat products on blood cholesterol.
Trends in Food Science and Technology 1992; 3: 137–141

3 Mermot M.
Editorial. The cholesterol papers
British Medical Journal 1994; 308: 351–352

4 Law M. R. and others
Systematic underestimation of association between serum cholesterol concentration and ischaemic heart disease in observational studies: data from the BUPA study.
British Medical Journal 1994; 308:363–366

5 Law M. R. and others
By how much and how quickly does reduction in serum cholesterol concentration lower risk of ischaemic heart disease?
British Medical Journal 1994; 308: 367–372

6 Law M. R. and others
Assessing possible hazards of reducing serum cholesterol.
British Medical Journal 1994; 308: 373–379

7 Gronbaek M. and others
Influence of sex, age, body mass index, and smoking on alcohol intake and mortality.
British Medical Journal 1994; 308: 303–307

8 Editorial. Inhibition of LDL oxidation by phenolic substances in red wine: a clue to the French paradox.
Nutrition Reviews 1993; 51 (6): 185–187

9 Frankel E. N. and others
Inhibition of oxidation of human low-density lipoproteins by phenolic substances in red wine.
Lancet 1993; 341: 454–457

10 Markovitz J. H. and others
Psychological predictors of hypertension in the Framingham Study: is there tension in hypertension?
Journal of the American Medical Association 1993; 270: 2439–2443

11 Pickering T. G.
Tension and hypertension.
Journal of the American Medical Association 1993; 270: 2494

12 Tang and others
How effective is nicotine replacement therapy in helping people to stop smoking?
British Medical Journal 1994; 308: 261–265

13 Andersson B. and others
The effects of exercise training on body composition and metabolism in men and women.
International Journal of Obesity 1991; 15: 75–81

14 Boyle K. and others
Waist to hip ratios in Australia: a different picture of obesity.
Australian Journal of Nutrition and Dietetics 1993; 50 (2)

15 Ball M. J. and others
Obesity and fat distribution in New Zealanders. A pattern of coronary heart disease risk.
New Zealand Medical Journal 1993; 106: 951

Dr. John Briffa, BSc (Hons) M.B. BS (Lond.), wrote chapters 2–4.

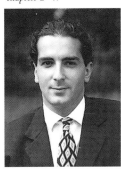

16 Lissner L. and others

Variability of body weight and health outcomes in the Framingham population.
New England Journal of Medicine
1991; 324: 1839–1844

17 Bouchard C.

Is weight fluctuation a risk factor?
New England Journal of Medicine
1991;324: 1887–1888

18 Whaley M. H. and others

Predictors of over- and under-estimation of age-predicted maximum heart rate.
Medicine and Science Sports and Exercise
1992; 24 (10): 1173–1179

19 Chen J. and others

Antioxidant status and cancer mortality in China.
International Journal of Epidemiology
1993; 21 (4): 625–631

20 Stocker R.

Antioxidants 'beneficial' but complicated.
Nutrition News 1993; 10: 2

21 Ainsleigh H. G.

Beneficial effects off sun exposure on cancer mortality.
Preventative Medicine 1993; 22: 132–140

22 May C. S. and others

Insulin dependent diabetes mellitus, physical activity and death.
American Journal of Epidemiology
1993; 137 (11): 74–81

23 Imperial Cancer
Research Fund GP Research Group

Effectiveness of a nicotine patch in helping people stop smoking: results of a randomized trial in general practice.
British Medical Journal 1993; 306: 1304–1308

24 Ireland P. and Giles G.

A review of diet and cancer: what are the prospects for prevention in Australia?
Cancer Forum (The Australian Cancer Society)
1993; 17 (2): 132–155

Booklets

1 **Allied Dunbar National Fitness Survey**

The Sports Council and the Health Education Authority 1992

2 **Dietary Guidelines
to Lower Your Cancer Risk**

World Cancer Research Fund

Books

1 *Nutritional Medicine*

Dr Stephen Davies and Dr Alan Stewart
Pan Books 1987

2 *Dine Out and Lose Weight*

Michael Montignac
Artulen 1991

3 *Optimum Nutrition*

Patrick Holford
ION Press 1992

4 *Nutrition Almanac*

Third Edition, Lavon J. Dunne
McGraw-Hill Publishers 1990

5 *Day Light Robbery*

Dr Damien Downing
Arrow Books 1988

6 *Nutrition for Sport*

Steve Wootton
Simon and Schuster 1988

7 *Learned Helplessness*

Martin Seligman
Random House NY 1992

Picture Acknowledgements